Common Bacterial Infections in Infancy and Childhood

Diagnosis and Treatment

Common Bacterial Infections in Infancy and Childhood

Diagnosis and Treatment

Edited by
M.I. Marks

McGill University. Montreal

MTPPRESS LIMITED *International Medical Publishers*

Common Bacterial Infections in Infancy and Childhood

Diagnosis and Treatment

Published in UK, Europe and Middle East
by MTP Press Limited
Falcon House
Lancaster
England

First Printing
ISBN 978-0-85200-509-5   ISBN 978-94-011-9653-6 (eBook)
DOI 10.1007/978-94-011-9653-6

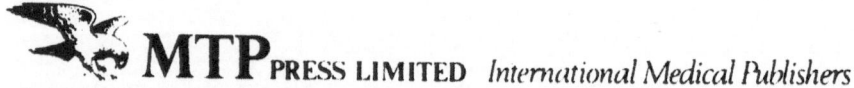

MTPPRESS LIMITED *International Medical Publishers*

Preface

Paediatrics is distinguished from general medicine by the different spectrum of disease encountered, and the interplay of disease and development within the growing child. Thus, clinical management taxes acumen, experience, and factual knowledge in a particularly challenging way. Infectious disease problems and their attendant pressures continue to dominate paediatric practice. As improvements in care approach marginal proportions, the onus on clinicians to provide prompt diagnosis and appropriate treatment gains increasing importance. Newcomers are often impressed by the pace of evolving syndromes, indicating the need for repeated examination and balanced judgement at all phases of illness.

This book considers common bacterial syndromes from a modern perspective. The authors' attitudes and opinions reflect their experience of paediatric infectious disease in a large teaching hospital. Thus, we are daily concerned with an overall minority of patients who fail to respond to domicilary measures, or who develop a specific complication. We believe this perspective will have particular relevance for community practitioners who take satisfaction in the care of sick children, and for house officers faced with the dual problems of an ill child and alarmed parents.

M.I. Marks
Montreal, January, 1979

Contributors

Ahronheim, Gerald A.
Assistant Professor of Paediatrics, McGill University, Montreal.

Marks, Melvin I.
Associate Professor of Paediatrics and Assistant Professor of Microbiology and Immunology, McGill University, Montreal.

Spratt, H. Clifford
Lecturer in Paediatrics, McGill University, Montreal.

Contents

Chapter 1

Principles of Antibacterial Therapy in Infants and Children

M.I. Marks

Chapter II

Respiratory Infections

H.C. Spratt, G.A. Ahronheim and M.I. Marks

Chapter III

Infections of the Central Nervous System

G.A. Ahronheim

Chapter IV

Genitourinary Infections

M.I. Marks

Chapter V

Skin and Wound Infections

M.I. Marks

Chapter VI

Infections of the Skeletal System

G.A. Ahronheim

Chapter VII

Enteric Infections

M.I. Marks

Chapter VIII

Neonatal Infections

H.C. Spratt

Chapter I

Principles of Antibacterial Therapy in Infants and Children

M.I. Marks

Treatment of bacterial infections of infants and children should be based on an understanding of the pathogenesis of disease and the pharmacology of the drugs prescribed. Although generalisations are often used to formulate guidelines for therapy, the complexities of host-parasite relationships frequently require individualisation of the therapeutic programme. In this chapter, rationales for the selection of antibiotics, and the choice of dose, route of administration and duration of treatment are provided. The scientific basis for these choices depends on knowledge of the cause and natural course of bacterial infections in the paediatric age group as outlined in the following chapters. We do not treat pneumonia, but rather the cause(s) of pneumonia in a particular host. Such treatment programmes may include antipyretics, nutritional therapy, and fluid, electrolyte and acid-base management as well. Surgical debridement, drainage, immobilisation and rest, and removal of foreign bodies may be the most critical components of certain treatment programmes. Careful explanations of rationale and directions to the patient and parents (where indicated) cannot be overemphasised. With these considerations in mind, I shall outline an approach to the choices involved in antibacterial therapy.

1. Factors Influencing the Selection of Antibacterial Drugs

1.1 Characteristics of Infection

How does the clinician select an antibacterial drug? The answer to this question involves a set of carefully learned responses that consider the cause of the particular infection and weigh the benefits and risks of the therapeutic agents available. For example, let us consider pharyngitis, an infection that may often not benefit from antibacterial therapy (Komaroff, 1978). If the clinical presentation includes features of the common cold syndrome (i.e. a history of exposure, rhinorrhoea, cough), the cause is usually a rhinovirus and antibiotics are not required. In such cases the cause is known, the benefits of antibiotics are negligible and, therefore, any risks are clearly unjustifiable.

However, if the patient has pharyngitis and anterior cervical lymphadenitis instead of the abovementioned signs, he may require antibacterial therapy for group A streptococcal infection. The clinical suspicion of streptococcal pharyngitis may be erroneous in up to 50 % of cases and, therefore, the clinician must use the laboratory to assist in the diagnosis (Peter and Smith, 1977). If we assume that the throat culture confirms the diagnosis of streptococcal pharyngitis, which drug do we choose? Perhaps, we should ask another question first: why should we prescribe a drug for this condition? In this situation, treatment may shorten the course of illness, may avert complications (such as suppurative lymphadenitis, sinusitis and, rarely, bacteraemia), and may prevent long term complications (e.g. rheumatic fever) [Kaplan et al., 1977a]. The latter benefit of drug therapy is a most important consideration and should be emphasised in discussion of the diagnosis and therapy with the patient and parents. My choice in this situation is penicillin V (phenoxymethylpenicillin) for the following reasons:

1) Penicillin V is resistant to acid degradation and, therefore, its absorption from the gastrointestinal tract is more complete.

2) Controlled evaluations have confirmed the efficacy of penicillin V in the prevention of rheumatic fever if the patient takes it for 10 days (Kaplan et al., 1977a).

3) Experience with this drug and its therapeutic, pharmacological and toxic properties extends over several decades. Children are rarely allergic to penicillin and the drug is inexpensive and reasonably palatable.

1.2 Drug Allergies

Hypersensitivity to antibiotics occurs occasionally in children and rarely in infants and newborns. The systemic and dermatological features of true allergic reactions consist of anaphylaxis, anaphylactoid reactions, urticaria, pruritic maculopapular exanthems, glossostomatitis, interstitial nephritis and serum sickness-like syndromes. These reactions should not be confused with non-pruritic macular or maculopapular rashes which are often viral in origin. Nor should headache, myalgia and other nonspecific complaints be accepted as evidence of drug allergy. A careful history is, therefore, essential. This history must be considered in the light of the indication for therapy, the route used and the alternatives available. Skin testing with penicilloyl-polylysine and minor determinant mixture of benzylpenicillin can be

Table I. Schedule for desensitisation to penicillin[1]

1.	Prepare adrenaline (epinephrine) 1:1,000 and equipment for respiratory support and blood pressure monitoring
2.	Inject 0.1ml of penicillin 1,000 units/ml intradermally
3.	If no wheal and flare (or systemic) reaction in 20 minutes, repeat intradermal injections with doubling concentrations until 64,000 units/ml dose
4.	Repeat step 3 by the subcutaneous route (from 1,000 to 64,000 units/ml)
5.	If no reaction, proceed with therapy under close supervision

1 NB. Rarely necessary due to the increasing availability of alternative antibiotics.

employed to confirm penicillin hypersensitivity and to partially exclude the likelihood of immediate reactions (Warrington et al., 1978). Unfortunately, it cannot predict which patients will have delayed reactions.

Minor infections in normal hosts, such as streptococcal pharyngitis and impetigo, rarely require parenteral therapy. A child with a history of penicillin-associated rash may be treated with erythromycin. Cephalosporins (e.g. cephalexin) can be substituted for penicillin in the treatment of staphylococcal furunculosis; however, there is some degree of cross-reactivity between these two drug classes and allergic reactions to cephalosporins may occur in 10 to 20% of patients allergic to penicillin. The oral route appears to decrease the severity of these reactions; furthermore, anaphylaxis rarely occurs with this route. In the exceptional case where it has occurred, its onset is within the first 45 minutes. It is a wise precaution, therefore, to have the allergic patient wait for this time period after the first oral dose of medication.

In more severe infections, one must often choose between more toxic alternative drugs or desensitisation procedures. For example, chloramphenicol should be employed for the therapy of epiglottitis, arthritis and meningitis due to *Haemophilus influenzae* when the patient is allergic to penicillin (since all the penicillins are cross-allergenic). In other situations, laboratory evaluation of the activity of drug combinations can be used to guide therapy. We have found co-trimoxazole, erythromycin/rifampicin, and co-trimoxazole/rifampicin very useful in life-threatening infections in allergic patients or where conventional drug therapy is inappropriate for other reasons. However, caution is urged in the use of these combinations in patients. Laboratory testing to rule out antagonism and a careful review of the properties of the drug to avoid incompatibilities and cumulative toxicities are important first steps.

If judged essential, desensitisation to penicillin can be carried out by a series of inoculations as outlined in table I. This procedure is slow and painful, and rarely indicated in children.

Table II. Selection of antibacterial agents for specific bacterial pathogens (NB. Laboratory studies may suggest better choices in certain cases)

Bacteria	First choice	Second choice
Acinetobacter	Gentamicin	Kanamycin
Actinomyces	Penicillin	Erythromycin
Bacillus	Penicillin	Erythromycin
Bacteroides spp.	Chloramphenicol	Metronidazole
Bordetella pertussis	Erythromycin	Ampicillin (amoxycillin)
Borrelia	Tetracycline	Chloramphenicol
Brucella	Tetracycline ± streptomycin	Co-trimoxazole
Campylobacter fetus	Gentamicin	Tetracycline
Clostridium spp.	Penicillin	Erythromycin
Corynebacterium diphtheriae	Erythromycin	Penicillin
Enterobacter	Gentamicin	Ampicillin (amoxycillin)
Erysipelothrix	Penicillin	Tetracycline
Escherichia coli	Gentamicin[1]	Ampicillin (amoxycillin)[2]
Francisella tularensis	Streptomycin	Tetracycline
Haemophilus influenzae	Ampicillin (amoxycillin)	Chloramphenicol
Klebsiella	Gentamicin	Cephalosporin
Legionnaire's bacterium	Erythromycin	Rifampicin
Leptospira spp.	Ampicillin (amoxycillin)	Penicillin or Tetracycline
Listeria	Ampicillin (amoxycillin)	Penicillin
Mima, Moraxella	Gentamicin	Tetracycline
Mycobacterium tuberculosis	Isoniazid + rifampicin	Ethambutol + streptomycin
Mycobacterium, atypical	Isoniazid + rifampicin	Ethambutol + isoniazid
		Rifampicin + erythromycin
Mycobacterium marinum	Minocycline	Isoniazid + rifampicin
Mycobacterium leprae	Dapsone ± rifampicin	Clofazimine + dapsone
Mycoplasma pneumoniae	Erythromycin	Tetracycline
Neisseria gonorrhoeae	Penicillin	Ampicillin (amoxycillin)
		or spectinomycin
Neisseria meningitidis	Penicillin	Chloramphenicol
Nocardia	Co-trimoxazole	Trisulphapyrimidines
Pasteurella multocida	Penicillin	Tetracycline
Proteus mirabilis	Gentamicin	Ampicillin (amoxycillin)
Proteus spp.	Gentamicin	Carbenicillin or chloramphenicol
Providencia	Kanamycin	Ampicillin (amoxycillin)
Pseudomonas aeruginosa	Gentamicin ± carbenicillin	Carbenicillin or amikacin
Salmonella typhi	Co-trimoxazole or chloramphenicol	Ampicillin
Salmonella spp.	Ampicillin (amoxycillin)	Co-trimoxazole
Serratia	Gentamicin	Chloramphenicol
Shigella	Ampicillin	Co-trimoxazole
Spirillum minus	Penicillin	Erythromycin
Staphylococcus (β-lactamase positive)	Cloxacillin	Cephalosporin

Table II. (continued)

Staphylococcus (β-lactamase negative)	Penicillin	Erythromycin
Streptococcus (pyogenes, pneumoniae, viridans)	Penicillin	Erythromycin
Streptococcus, Group B	Penicillin	Chloramphenicol
Streptococcus faecalis	Penicillin + streptomycin[3]	Ampicillin (amoxycillin) + gentamicin
Streptococcus bovis	Penicillin	Erythromycin
Treponema pallidum	Penicillin	Erythromycin
Yersinia enterocolitica	Co-trimoxazole	Kanamycin
Yersinia pestis	Streptomycin	Chloramphenicol

1 Preferred choice for sepsis and other infections.
2 Preferred choice for urinary tract infections. Sulphonamides may also be useful.
3 In endocarditis.

1.3 Susceptibility of Bacteria

Table II lists drug choices for common bacterial causes of infection. This table is derived from *in vitro* tests of susceptibility which are usually correlated with *in vivo* evaluations. For example, it is not difficult to eradicate *Streptococcus pneumoniae* or *Neisseria meningitidis* with antibiotics to which they are sensitive *in vitro;* however, this is not always the case. The efficacy of any particular antibacterial agent is also related to the site of infection and the distribution of the drug. For example, benzathine penicillin G may reach adequate levels in the serum but not the CSF, making this drug inappropriate for the treatment of congenital syphilis (Speer et al., 1977). As a consequence, sensitive bacteria may persist in the leptomeninges and cerebrospinal fluid despite *in vitro* sensitivity. Other reasons for failure of antibacterial therapy include host factors, such as neutropenia, immune deficiencies, cystic fibrosis, poor activity of the drug at the site of infection (e.g. due to a pH effect or inhibitors in pus), incompatible mixtures, antagonistic combinations and inappropriate route of administration (e.g. chloramphenicol by the intramuscular route) [Dupont et al., 1970]. Walled-off abscesses, necrotic tissue, foreign bodies and facultative intracellular parasites (e.g. Brucella, Listeria, tubercle bacilli) may also create situations where the *in vivo* activity of antibacterial drugs is markedly reduced. Of course, poor compliance may be the most obvious reason for failure (Rabinovitch et al., 1973).

Reasons for apparent discrepancies between *in vitro* sensitivity tests and actual clinical results should be sought in the laboratory as well. The difficulties of accurately measuring sensitivities of *H. influenzae* and of testing drugs such as co-trimoxazole are recent examples of laboratory pitfalls (Marks and Weinmaster, 1975). Commonly employed sensitivity tests use the disc diffusion, broth dilution or agar dilution methods; enzyme activity (i.e. β-lactamase) is often used to examine penicillin

Table III. Antibacterial drugs that may induce haemolysis in patients with glucose-6-phosphate dehydrogenase (G6PD) deficiency

Chloramphenicol	Nitrofurantoin
Co-trimoxazole	Para-aminosalicylic acid (PAS)
Isoniazid	Sulphonamides
Nalidixic acid	

sensitivity. Readers are referred to other sources for details of these methods (e.g. Braude, 1976), but it suffices to say that each of these tests requires carefully standardised methods, use of controls and periodic quality evaluation. The disc test for meningococcal susceptibility, for example, must pay strict attention to the media and type of sulphonamide disc used (Hammerberg et al., 1976). Clinicians would be well advised to familiarise themselves with these tests and to take an occasional refresher period in the laboratory they work with most often. A generous dose of sincere questioning is the best stimulus for most laboratory directors. Modern infectious disease services assume this role in many university teaching centres.

1.4 Patient Age

The choice of antibacterial drugs in newborns and children is limited by age-related toxicities. For example, in the newborn, sulphonamides compete with bilirubin for albumin binding and kernicterus may result. The common presence of hyperbilirubinaemia (often due to immature hepatic enzymes) and the peculiar permeability of the blood brain barrier in the newborn are responsible. The tetracyclines are deposited in developing teeth and bones of children up to eight years of age and can cause a brownish discolouration of the enamel as well as some skeletal growth impairment (Grossman, 1971); the risk of this is greatest the earlier in life the exposure occurs, including the intrauterine period. The newborn's immature liver may also compound the effects of certain drug interactions such as that between phenytoin and chloramphenicol so that toxic concentrations may be reached even though conventional neonatal doses have been given (Riley, 1972; Rose et al., 1977).

Antibacterial therapy of newborns often needs to be initiated well before laboratory confirmation of infection and bacterial susceptibility are available. The principles governing the choice of drugs in this situation are outlined in chapter VIII on neonatal bacterial infection. These include knowledge of the susceptibility patterns of the pathogenic bacterial flora in the nursery, features of the mother's condition in the peripartum period, and familiarity with the pharmacology of antibacterial drugs in newborns. The pharmacokinetics of several regimens (ampicillin and gentamicin, cephalothin and tobramycin, ampicillin and amikacin) have been described and appear to be safe as well as active against the majority of paediatric pathogens (Marks et al., 1978). These or alternative regimens can be used on a rotating schedule in response to changes in nursery bacterial resistance patterns.

Table IV. Major toxicities of antibacterial drugs

Drug	Major toxicities				
	Gastro-intestinal	Haema-tological	Hepatic	Vestibulo-auditory	Renal
Aminoglycosides[1]				+	+
Cephaloridine (high doses)					+
Chloramphenicol		+			
Clindamycin/lincomycin	+				
Co-trimoxazole		+			
Erythromycin estolate			+		
Nitrofurantoin[2]	+				
Para-aminosalicylic acid	+				
Penicillins	+				
Penicillins (methicillin)					+
Polymyxins					+
Rifampicin		+	+		
Sulphonamides		+			
Tetracyclines	+				+[3]
Tetracyclines (minocycline)				+	

1   Includes gentamicin, tobramycin, amikacin, kanamycin, streptomycin and neomycin.

2   Pulmonary reactions and peripheral neuropathy (with high blood levels e.g. in presence of renal failure) are also important toxic effects of nitrofurantoin.

3   May aggravate pre-existing azotaemia and uraemia (not due to nephrotoxicity *per se* but rather the antianabolic effect of tetracyclines). Risk less with doxycycline.

1.5 Other Host Factors

Patients with glucose-6-phosphate dehydrogenase (G6PD) deficiency are prone to haemolytic episodes with certain antibacterials. These drugs are listed in table III and should be avoided in these subjects. Drugs such as chloramphenicol which have a marked tendency to cause haematological complications, should not be used in patients with pre-existing bone marrow suppression. This principle also applies to hepatotoxic and nephrotoxic drugs in patients with pre-existing liver and kidney disease, respectively. A list of the major toxicities of antibacterial drugs is provided in table IV.

1.6 Bacteriostatic or Bactericidal Drugs?

The type and site of infection often guide the choice of drug. For example, erythromycin and the cephalosporins are not useful for the treatment of meningitis, and bacteriostatic drugs are rarely effective in endocarditis. A list of bacteriostatic and bactericidal drugs is presented in table V. It should be remembered that these designa-

Table V. Mechanisms of action of antibacterial drugs[1]

Mechanism of action	Bactericidal drugs	Bacteriostatic drugs
Cell wall inhibitors (prevent cell wall synthesis)	Penicillins Cephalosporins Vancomycin Bacitracin	
Cell membrane inhibitors (injure cell membrane)	Polymyxins	
Protein synthesis inhibitors (bind to bacterial ribosomes)	Aminoglycosides[2]	Tetracyclines Chloramphenicol Macrolides[3]
Nucleic acid inhibitors a) inhibit nucleic acid synthesis	Rifampicin	
b) block uptake and formation of essential metabolites by cell		Sulphonamides Trimethoprim Para-aminosalicylic acid (PAS) Sulphones

1   NB. A drug's ability to kill or inhibit bacteria can vary under certain circumstances, such as combinations of drugs or against specific pathogens.
2   Includes gentamicin, tobramycin, amikacin, kanamycin, streptomycin and neomycin.
3   Includes erythromycin, clindamycin and lincomycin.

tions are not absolute; for example, penicillins may only inhibit the growth of certain strains of staphylococci (Peterson et al., 1978), and chloramphenicol may kill Haemophilus very efficiently (Turk, 1977). Other drugs are more active in combination (e.g. sulphonamides and trimethoprim) than alone.

Certain characteristics of the host may suggest the need for bactericidal drugs. Children with immune deficiencies, particularly of the opsonophagocytic defense mechanisms, fall into this category. These include neutropenic leukaemia patients, and those with hypogammaglobulinaemia and true or functional asplenia. For example, treatment of Salmonella infections in a patient with marked splenic dysfunction due to sickle cell anaemia should be with bactericidal antibiotics.

1.7 Indications for Prophylactic Antibacterial Therapy

The principle that non-bacterial infections (e.g. varicella, parainfluenza croup, etc.) should not be treated with antibacterial drugs is worth repeating. Similarly, antibacterial drugs are not ordinarily justified to prevent bacterial complications of viral disease such as influenza or bronchiolitis. There is no question they are indicated in the *treatment* of these complications however, and they should be prescribed as early in the course of infection as possible. The skills of the clinician are essential in the application of these principles to human disease. Therein lies the art and many rewards of clinical medicine.

Prophylactic antibacterial drugs have a useful role in the prevention of wound infections, in contaminated gastrointestinal surgery such as appendectomy (Foster and O'Toole, 1978) in endocarditis, and in the prevention of recurrences of rheumatic fever and urinary tract infections. Their usefulness in the prevention of asplenic bacteraemia, post-traumatic meningitis and infections after many surgical procedures, is less obvious. A list of indications and suggested drug choices for antibacterial prophylaxis is provided in table VI.

Table VI. Indications for prophylactic antibacterial therapy

Prevention of	Drug(s) of choice
Endocarditis (Kaplan et al., 1977b):	
a) With dental procedures and upper respiratory tract surgery	Penicillin
b) With genitourinary and gastrointestinal tract surgery	Ampicillin + gentamicin
c) With cardiovascular surgery	Cloxacillin
Gonococcal ophthalmia	1% silver nitrate solution or erythromycin ointment
Meningococcal infection	Rifampicin or sulphonamide (strain must be susceptible; for sulphonamide resistance use minocycline if unable to use rifampicin)
Rheumatic fever	Penicillin
Urinary tract infection	
a) Chronic recurrent	Nitrofurantoin or co-trimoxazole
b) With catheter drainage	Irrigation with neomycin + polymyxin
c) With urogenital surgery in patients with positive urine cultures	As indicated by *in vitro* studies
Wound infection — gastrointestinal surgery	Cephalosporins or ampicillin + gentamicin

2. Factors Influencing Dosage

2.1 Characteristics of Infection

The correct dose of an antibacterial drug is that which ensures its optimal concentration at the site of infection. The optimal concentration is often in the range of 4 to 8 times the minimum inhibitory concentration (MIC) of the drug, but can occasionally be as low as 2 to 4 times the MIC. Local factors such as pH, the presence of purulent and inflammatory fluids, the presence of leucocytes and redox potential may all affect drug activity. Therefore, tests of antibacterial activity in body fluids (e.g. serum, CSF, urine, synovial fluid, etc.) may be very appropriate guides to optimal dosage recommendation. Concentrations of each drug may vary considerably at different sites. For example, the dose of ampicillin chosen for *H. influenzae* meningitis is usually 200 to 400mg/kg/day in order to overcome a relatively low CSF/serum ratio, whereas urinary tract infections (where the drug reaches high concentrations) may often be effectively treated with 50 to 100mg/kg/day. Such dosage adjustments are of benefit in reducing dose-related side effects, such as diarrhoea, electrolyte overload, convulsions, haematological suppression, etc., as well as being economical.

Specific dosage recommendations for various infections are included in the text and tables in the following chapters.

2.2 Susceptibility of Bacteria

An often asked question is: 'What is the dose of . . . ?'; usually, that dose that provides reasonable drug concentrations with a margin of safety for the patient. In supplying the conventional dosage recommendations, however, it is important to emphasise that these apply only to patients with normal metabolic and excretory functions and to infections caused by common pathogenic bacteria in a site easily reached by the antibacterial drug in question. If these criteria are not met, and/or the therapeutic:toxic ratio for the drug in question is narrow for this patient, consideration should be given to individualisation of the dosage.

The next step, after the choice of a drug, is the susceptibility of the infecting bacteria. The disc diffusion tests in common usage in clinical laboratories do not supply quantitative results. They can only divide bacteria into sensitive and resistant populations. Agar dilution, tube dulution and gradient plate methods etc. can be used to accurately measure the concentration of drug necessary to inhibit or kill specific bacteria *in vitro;* this can usually be measured only indirectly *in vivo.* For example, the serum inhibitory power (i.e. the highest dilution of the patient's serum that will still inhibit the growth of the bacteria causing the infection) usually associated with the successful management of endocarditis is 1:8 (Klastersky et al., 1974). More stringent criteria have proven successful for less well vascularised infections, e.g. a

Table VII. Major pathways of elimination (excretion/metabolism) of antibacterial drugs

Renal:	*Hepato-biliary:*	*Other:*
Aminoglycosides[1]	Chloramphenicol	Doxycycline
Cephalosporins	Doxycycline	Macrolides[3]
Nitrofurantoin	Isoniazid	
Penicillins	Macrolides[3]	
Polymyxins	Minocycline	
Sulphonamides	Rifampicin	
Tetracyclines[2]		
Trimethoprim		

1 Includes gentamicin, tobramycin, amikacin, kanamycin, streptomycin and neomycin.
2 Except minocycline.
3 Includes erythromycin, clindamycin and lincomycin.

serum *killing* power of 1:8 for skeletal infections (Tetzlaff et al., 1978). Although similar figures are not available for meningitis, the antibacterial ability of the CSF can also be used to guide dosage. Titration of body fluid antibacterial concentrations against the sensitivity of the infecting bacteria (with knowledge of the toxic levels of the drug) can be attempted.

On the basis of these findings, alterations in dosage may be necessary. Alternatively, drugs that block renal excretion (e.g. probenecid) could be used to increase serum concentrations without increasing the dose (e.g. with the penicillins or cephalosporins where large oral doses increase the risk of gastrointestinal upset).

The quantitative susceptibility of bacteria can also be altered by combinations of drugs. For example, conventional doses of carbenicillin and gentamicin may be active against Pseudomonas when administered together, but inactive when prescribed alone. A note of caution here: these two drugs should not be mixed in the same intravenous solution as they may be inactivated in this way (Riff and Jackson, 1972). Tests of synergy are useful in predicting these activities in the laboratory and should precede the use of novel drug combinations in patients. This is so because combinations also have the potential for antagonism. More exact tests of drug-bacteria interaction (e.g. rate of killing) may provide even more specific guidelines for dosage recommendations in the future.

2.3 Patient Age

Dosages in the newborn are characteristically lower, and the interval between administration longer, than those recommended for older children — e.g. 25mg/kg/day for chloramphenicol and 50,000u/kg/day (administered 12-hourly) for penicillin in the first week of life (McCracken and Nelson, 1977). This is based on the presence of immature liver conjugating enzyme systems for chloramphenicol and a decreased renal excretion rate for penicillin. Thus, knowledge of the pathways of drug excretion and metabolism and the influence of age on these mechanisms, are critical for proper dosage selection (table VII).

2.4 Other Host Factors

Patients with liver or kidney disease are similar to newborns in that dosage frequencies must be adjusted in keeping with the estimated half-life of the drug administered. This is particularly difficult to estimate when function is changing. Serial measurements of serum concentrations are essential in such situations. These results must be interpreted in the light of the known quantitative susceptibility of the offending pathogen and the site of infection. More rapid microbiological, enzymatic and radionuclide methods are becoming available for this purpose. The objectives are to achieve a peak serum activity above the MIC of the bacteria and to maintain a peak and trough level below that recognised to cause toxicity. An example is illustrated in figure 1. Theoretical properties of this 'ideal' drug include rapid absorption, large therapeutic:toxic ratio, no accumulation, constant half-life and high activity against susceptible bacteria.

Occasionally, hosts may have accelerated metabolic or excretory functions that can lower antibacterial concentrations to subtherapeutic levels. For example, patients

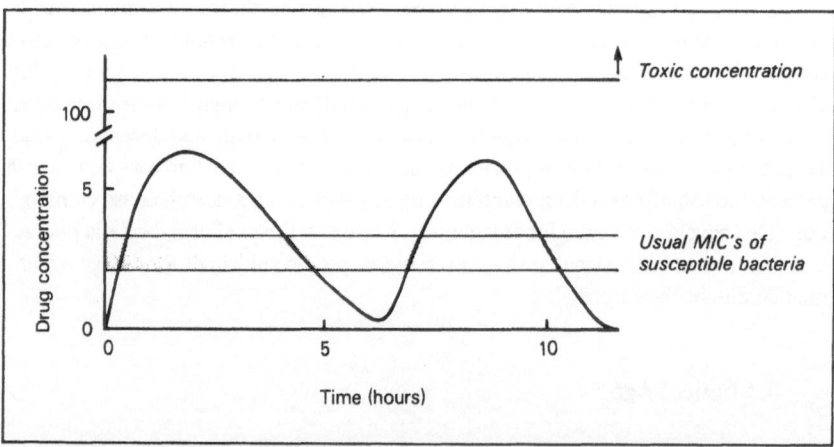

Fig. 1. Pharmacological properties of the 'ideal' antibacterial agent. Drug concentrations surpass the usual MIC's of the infecting bacteria at the site of infection and are well below the concentrations toxic to mammalian cells. Additional advantages include a predictable and reasonable half-life, without accumulation.

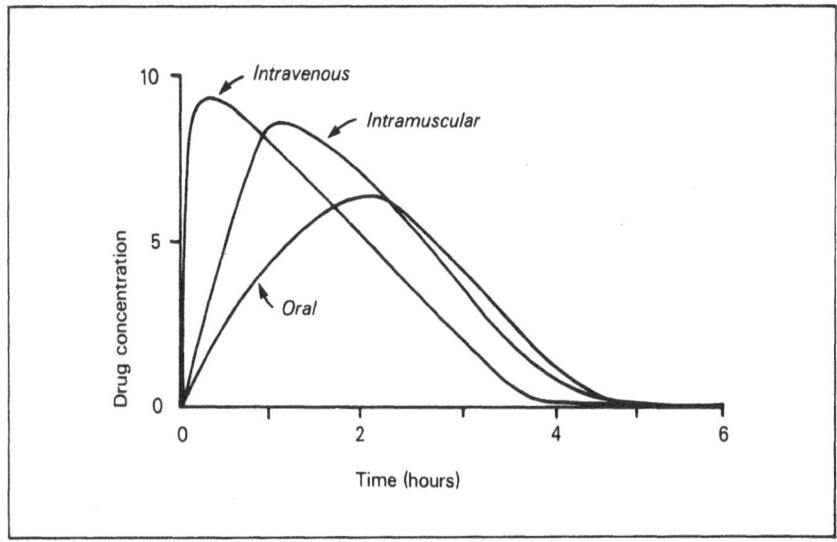

Fig. 2. Theoretical serum concentrations of an antibacterial agent administered by 3 different routes (intravenous given over 15 minutes). Oral antibacterial agents actually vary considerably in the speed and degree of absorption. This may depend on the drug (e.g. the absorption of chloramphenicol is excellent while that of benzathine penicillin is poor), or its form (e.g. suspensions are usually more rapidly absorbed than capsules or tablets).

receiving phenobarbitone may have lowered levels of chloramphenicol due to induction of liver enzymes (Palmer et al., 1972). Some patients with cystic fibrosis seem to have increased renal excretory mechanisms for penicillins such as methicillin and dicloxacillin, thereby lowering serum concentrations (Jusko et al., 1975; Yaffe et al., 1977). It is likely, therefore, that sputum concentrations (which probably depend on diffusion of drug from the serum) are also lowered and the antistaphylococcal effects of these drugs are much poorer than expected.

3. Factors Influencing the Choice of Route

The choice of route depends on many of the same principles outlined above. These include consideration of the pharmacology of the drug (figure 2), the site of infection and the quantitative susceptibility of the infecting bacteria. Properties of certain antibacterials prevent their use by one or more routes. These properties include poor absorption, acid lability, pain on injection and toxicity (e.g. nitrofurantoin parenterally). These are summarised in table VIII. Some drugs are useful because of superior absorption by the oral route and in most situations offer no advantage over conventional therapy when used parenterally. Amoxycillin (Marks and Vose, 1978) is an example of this.

Table VIII. Routes to be avoided with certain antibacterial drugs[1]

Oral (poor absorption)	Intramuscular	Intravenous
Aminoglycosides	Carbenicillin (painful)	Indanyl carbenicillin (carindacillin)
'Parenteral' cephalosporins:	Cephalothin (painful)	Erythromycin
cephalothin	Chloramphenicol	(rarely indicated)
cephaloridine	(erratic absorption)	Nitrofurantoin
cephamandole	Nitrofurantoin	Procaine penicillin
cephazolin	Vancomycin (painful)	
'Parenteral' penicillins:		
benzathine penicillin		
procaine penicillin		
carbenicillin		
methicillin		
ticarcillin		
Polymyxins		
Vancomycin		

1   See text for exceptions.

3.1 Indications for Oral Therapy

Oral therapy is obviously impossible in comatose patients and those with vomiting or obstructing gastrointestinal lesions. Without monitoring of absorption, distribution and *in vivo* efficacy, oral therapy is unreliable in many serious invasive infections. This is particularly true with antibacterial drugs that are absorbed only moderately well by the oral route (e.g. oral penicillins and oral cephalosporins). Some drugs, such as chloramphenicol, are absorbed so well by mouth that this route is often used for the treatment of serious infections such as typhoid fever. Monitoring in certain patients (e.g. newborns) may still be necessary, however, since metabolism may be variable (Black et al., 1978). Others, of course, are not absorbed by this route and should not be used for the therapy of extragastrointestinal infections (e.g. aminoglycosides, polymyxins, methicillin, cephalothin).

There are specific indications for oral therapy. For example, gastrointestinal infections due to enteropathogenic *E. coli* seem to respond best to oral colistin or neomycin with little risk to the patient (Nelson, 1971). Oral therapy may be useful as an adjunct to parenteral therapy of systemic infections that also involve the gastrointestinal tract (e.g. enterocolitis and septicaemia), and it also has a role in preoperative bowel preparation and hepatic coma. However, oral therapy may alter gastrointestinal bacterial flora to the detriment of the patient (e.g. loss of vitamin K producing bacteria, *Candida albicans* superinfections, and pseudomembranous colitis).

With efficient and careful monitoring, oral therapy has been used successfully for the therapy of endocarditis, osteomyelitis and septic arthritis (Nelson et al., 1978;

Tetzlaff et al., 1978). This is an important trend in chemotherapy, significant for its reduction in the need for parenteral therapy and hospitalisation and their attendant risks (e.g. nosocomial infections, psychological trauma). Careful follow-up for monitoring of effective serum concentrations and tests of compliance are essential to this approach.

3.2 Indications for Intramuscular Therapy

Intramuscular antibacterial therapy should be reserved for drugs that are poorly absorbed by the oral route (table VIII) and where intravenous therapy is not practical. The intramuscular route does provide higher blood concentrations more rapidly than oral administration (figure 2), and is very useful for the administration of aminoglycosides to newborns (McCracken and Nelson, 1977). Intramuscular therapy is often used for rheumatic fever prophylaxis (e.g. benzathine penicillin) particularly in situations where compliance is poor by the oral route (Breese et al., 1965). It must be remembered, however, that these injections are painful for these children and in themselves are often responsible for poor compliance and reluctance to return for follow-up examinations. It is not unusual to notice a transient limp due to gluteal muscle pain or, occasionally, due to injury to the sciatic nerve.

Allergic reactions are most difficult to treat after intramuscular injection, particularly with long-acting preparations such as benzathine penicillin. Fibrosis and strictures of the quadriceps muscles and gangrene of the foot have been reported after multiple injections of aminoglycosides in newborns (Talbert et al., 1967). Care must be exercised in avoiding intravascular injection of procaine penicillin. Of course, the intramuscular route is contraindicated in patients with disorders of coagulation.

Sterile abscesses (often very painful) have been produced by large intramuscular injections of several antibacterial drugs including ampicillin. It is my opinion that intramuscular therapy is a poor substitute for the extra time and care needed from health professionals to ensure compliance by direct observation of oral ingestion, by careful explanation of the course of illness and benefit of therapy, and by judicious follow-up and monitoring of oral antibacterial therapy. It should never be a substitute for intravenous therapy in the patient in shock and should not be used for the convenience of the clinician.

3.3 Indications for Intravenous Therapy

The intravenous route is essential for the treatment of infected comatose patients and for those in shock. This route is reasonably painless once the small scalp vein needle is securely positioned and is often preferred by children instead of periodic painful intramuscular injections. Intravenous therapy may be necessary for hydra-

Table IX. Incompatibilities and drug interactions with commonly prescribed antibacterial drugs

Antibacterial drug	Incompatibilities and drug interactions
Ampicillin	Incompatible with alkaline solutions; hyperalimentation solutions; 5% glucose and water
Carbenicillin	Incompatible with gentamicin/kanamycin or colistin (in same solution); amino acid solutions
Cephalothin	Incompatible with polymyxins/tetracycline/erythromycin/calcium
Chloramphenicol	Incompatible with polymyxins/tetracycline/vancomycin/hydrocortisone/vitamin B/alcohol May increase serum levels of phenytoin Phenobarbitone may decrease serum levels of chloramphenicol
Clindamycin	Incompatible with vitamin B
Co-trimoxazole	Additive antifolate effect with pyrimethamine and methotrexate
Gentamicin	Incompatible with heparin/penicillins (in same solution) Increased risk of ototoxicity when combined with ethacrynic acid, or frusemide in renal failure
Isoniazid	Antacids may reduce absorption May increase serum phenytoin levels
Kanamycin	See gentamicin Unstable in hyperalimentation solutions
Penicillins	Incompatible with amphotericin B/metaraminol/phenylephrine/tetracycline/vancomycin/vitamin C/bisulphite (in same solution); acid pH
Methicillin	Incompatible with tetracycline/kanamycin
Nafcillin	Incompatible with vitamin B
Rifampicin	Serum levels may be decreased by simultaneous PAS May decrease serum levels of corticosteroids Phenobarbitone may decrease serum levels of rifampicin
Sulphonamides	May increase serum levels of phenytoin (sulphaphenazole; ?sulphamethizole) May increase activity of methotrexate
Vancomycin	Incompatible with chloramphenicol/heparin/hydrocortisone/penicillin

tion, alimentation, etc. and this may provide a convenient route for antibacterial therapy. It is a source of amazement to see intramuscular therapy administered to a child with a functioning intravenous line in place.

The speed with which high serum concentrations are attained with intravenous therapy is unsurpassed (figure 2). However, incompatibilities of antibacterial drugs with other therapies, chemicals, pH, etc., must be remembered when these drugs are mixed in intravenous solutions (table IX).

Intravenous therapy often requires hospitalisation and this may limit the patient's activities. There are ways of reducing these inconveniences, such as the use of 'heparin lock' systems that allow almost full mobility for the patient between infusion times. Intravenous infusions may be given rapidly (over 1 to 5 minutes) for most antibacterial drugs such as the penicillins and cephalosporins, but more slowly for the aminoglycosides, where the risk of neuromuscular blockade and respiratory arrest accompanies bolus injections. In all cases however, host characteristics (e.g. age, size, renal and/or hepatic function and electrolyte status) need to be considered in guiding the speed of infusion and choice of preparation. When in doubt, longer infusion times should be employed.

Intravenous therapy does increase the risk of nosocomial infection due to contaminated infusion material and/or infusion apparatus such as the needle or catheter (Zinner et al., 1969). The use of indwelling intravenous catheters (installed percutaneously or by cut-down) markedly increases this risk and should be avoided if possible. If they are used, the ideal is to place these catheters in peripheral veins under sterile conditions and to change the site every 72 hours, or earlier if signs of inflammation appear.

4. Factors Influencing the Duration of Treatment

There are very few prospective controlled studies of the optimal duration of antibacterial therapy. An exception is the treatment of group A streptococcal pharyngitis to prevent rheumatic fever. Here 10 days of penicillin therapy was clearly superior to 5 days. We have found that 7 days' therapy eradicates the bacteria as effectively as 10 days but could not test the probability that these two durations of therapy would be comparable in the prevention of rheumatic fever (Rabinovitch et al., 1973). Most of the other recommendations about duration are based upon clinical experience and careful retrospective observation. Critical factors involve some of the previously mentioned principles about the nature of the infecting bacteria, the site of infection and the immune competence of the host. Thus, superficial infections by common pathogens in normal hosts improve with very short (sometimes none) antibacterial treatment courses (e.g. 2 to 5 days), while endocarditis, osteomyelitis and neonatal meningitis due to similar bacteria may relapse if therapy is discontinued before 3 weeks.

Table X. Guidelines for duration of antibacterial therapy

1. *Single dose*
   Cystitis[1]
   Gonococcal urethritis
   Primary syphilis (benzathine penicillin therapy)

2. *48 hours after bacteriological and clinical improvement*
   Furunculosis
   Localised wound infection
   Conjunctivitis
   Rhinitis
   E. coli enteritis

3. *One week after bacteriological and clinical improvement*
   Epiglotittis
   Otitis media
   Shigella enterocolitis
   Sinusitis
   Pneumonia
   Meningitis (except in newborns or abnormal hosts — see below)
   Urinary tract infection
   Streptococcal infections (10 days' course recommended)
   Congenital and secondary syphilis

4. *Two weeks after bacteriological and clinical improvement*
   Neonatal meningitis
   Invasive infections in immune deficient patients
   Septic arthritis
   Deep abscesses including staphylococcal empyema
   Infections with Brucella, Listeria, Salmonella

5. *Long-term therapy necessary*

Endocarditis:	4 to 6 weeks
Acute osteomyelitis:	6 weeks
Chronic osteomyelitis:	6 months
Tuberculosis:	1 year
Leprosy — tuberculoid:	1 year
Leprosy — lepromatous:	5 years

1 Unfortunately, cystitis is often difficult to differentiate from upper urinary tract infection which requires a longer duration of therapy (see chapter IV; section 2.6.1).

Several 'rules of thumb' are useful for common bacterial infections in normal hosts. Antibacterial therapy can usually be discontinued 48 hours after bacteriological and clinical improvement of localised superficial infections (e.g. furunculosis and wound infections), one week after these events in common invasive infections in normal hosts (e.g. meningitis, bacteraemia and pneumonia), and two weeks after invasive infections in abnormal hosts (e.g. neonatal meningitis, and bacteraemia in leukaemics). Certain infections, such as endocarditis and osteomyelitis, and certain bacteria such as mycobacteria, are exceptions to these rules and require longer durations of therapy. Others, such as bacterial cystitis and gonococcal urethritis may be treated with only one dose of drug. These suggestions for duration of antibacterial therapy are summarised in table X. Clinical and bacteriological monitoring provide the bases for these decisions. In addition, certain laboratory guidelines, such as erythrocyte sedimentation rate, radiographs and leucocyte count can also be useful.

Future trends in antibacterial therapy will include more exact measurements of bacterial susceptibility, better means of monitoring appropriateness of dosage and route and, it is hoped, improved methods for ensuring the sterilisation/cure status of the patient. These developments should allow the use of lower doses, potent combinations, oral ambulatory therapy programmes, and shorter durations of treatment with less risk of toxicity to the patient.

References

Black, S.B.; Levine, P. and Shinefield, R.: The necessity for monitoring chloramphenicol levels when treating neonatal meningitis. Journal of Pediatrics 92: 235 (1978).

Braude, A.I.: Antimicrobial drug therapy; in Smith (Ed) Major Problems in Internal Medicine, Vol. 8 (Saunders, London 1976).

Breese, B.B.; Disney, F.A. and Talpez, W.B.: Penicillin in streptococcal infections. Total dose and frequency of administration. American Journal of Diseases of Children 110: 125 (1965).

Dupont, H.L.; Hornick, R.B.; Weiss, C.F.; Snyder, M.J. and Woodward, T.E.: Evaluation of chloramphenicol acid succinate therapy of induced typhoid fever and Rocky Mountain spotted fever. New England Journal of Medicine 282: 53 (1970).

Foster, P.D. and O'Toole, R.D.: Primary appendectomy. The effect of prophylactic cephaloridine on postoperative wound infection. Journal of the American Medical Association 239: 1411 (1978).

Grossman, E.R.; Walchek, A. and Freedman, H.: Tetracyclines and permanent teeth: The relationship between dose and tooth color. Pediatrics 47: 567 (1971).

Hammerberg, S.; Marks, M.I. and Weinmaster, G.: Re-evaluation of the disc diffusion method for sulfonamide susceptibility testing of *Neisseria meningitides*. Antimicrobial Agents and Chemotherapy 10: 869 (1976).

Jusko, W.J.; Mosovitch, L.L.; Gerbracht, L.M.; Mattar, M.E. and Yaffe, S.J.: Enhanced renal excretion of dicloxacillin in patients with cystic fibrosis. Pediatrics 56: 1038 (1975).

Kaplan, E.L.; Bisno, A.; Derrick, W.; Facklam, R.; Gordis, L.; Honser, H.B.; Jackson, W.H.; Millard, D.; Shulman, S.T.; Taranta, A.V. and Wannamaker, L.W.: Prevention of rheumatic fever. Circulation 55: 223 (1977a).

Kaplan, E.L.; Anthony, B.F.; Bisno, A.; Durack, D.; Phil, D.; Houser, H.; Millard, H.D.; Sanford, J.; Shulman, S.T.; Stillerman, M.; Taranta, A. and Wenger, N.: Prevention of bacterial endocarditis. Circulation 56: 139A (1977b).

Klastersky, J.; Daneau, D.; Swings, G. and Weerts, D.: Antibacterial activity in serum and urine as a therapeutic guide in bacterial infections. Journal of Infectious Diseases 129: 187 (1974).

Komaroff, A.L.: A management strategy for sore throat. Journal of the American Medical Association 239: 1429 (1978).

Marks, M.I. and Weinmaster, G.: Influences of media and inocula on the *in vitro* susceptibility of *Hemophilus influenzae* to co-trimoxazole, ampicillin, penicillin and chloramphenicol. Antimicrobial Agents and Chemotherapy 8: 657 (1975).

Marks, S.; Marks, M.I.; Dupont, C. and Hammerberg, S.: Evaluation of three antibiotic programs in newborn infants. Canadian Medical Association Journal 118: 659 (1978).

Marks, M.I. and Vose, A.D.: Evaluation of amoxicillin therapy in ill children. Journal of Clinical Pharmacology 18: 61 (1978).

McCracken, G.H. Jr. and Nelson, J.D.: in Antimicrobial Therapy for Newborns: Practical Application of Pharmacology to Clinical Usage (Grune & Stratton, London 1977).

Nelson, J.D.: Duration of neomycin therapy for enteropathogenic *Escherichia coli* diarrheal disease: A comparative study of 113 cases. Pediatrics 48: 248 (1971).

Nelson, J.D.; Howard, J.B. and Shelton, S.: Oral antibiotic therapy for skeletal infections of children. I. Antibiotic concentrations in suppurative synovial fluid. Journal of Pediatrics 92: 131 (1978).

Palmer, D.L.; Despopoulos, A. and Rael, E.D.: Induction of chloramphenicol metabolism by phenobarbital. Antimicrobial Agents and Chemotherapy 1: 112 (1972).

Peter, G. and Smith, A.L.: Group A streptococcal infections of the skin and pharynx. New England Journal of Medicine 297: 311 (1977).

Peterson, L.R.; Gerding, D.N.; Hall, W.H. and Schierl, E.A.: Medium-dependent variation in bactericidal activity of antibiotics against susceptible *Staphylococcus aureus*. Antimicrobial Agents and Chemotherapy 13: 665 (1978).

Rabinovitch, M.; Mackenzie, R.; Brazeau, M. and Marks, M.I.: Treatment of streptococcal pharyngitis. I. Clinical evaluation. Canadian Medical Association Journal 108: 1271 (1973).

Riff, L.J. and Jackson, G.G.: Laboratory and clinical conditions for gentamicin inactivation by carbenicillin. Archives of Internal Medicine 130: 887 (1972).

Riley, H.D. Jr.: Interactions among antimicrobial and nonantimicrobial agents. Pediatrics 50: 954 (1972).

Rose, J.Q.; Choi, H.K.; Schentag, J.J.; Kinkel, W.R. and Jusko, W.J.: Intoxication caused by interaction of chloramphenicol and phenytoin. Journal of the American Medical Association 237: 2630 (1977).

Speer, M.E.; Taber, L.H.; Clark, D.B. and Rudolph, A.J.: Cerebrospinal fluid levels of benzathine penicillin G in the neonate. Journal of Pediatrics 91: 996 (1977).

Talbert, J.L.; Haslam, R.H.A. and Haller, J.A. Jr.: Gangrene of the foot following intramuscular injection in the lateral thigh: A case report with recommendation for prevention. Journal of Pediatrics 70: 110 (1967).

Tetzlaff, T.R.; McCracken, G.H. Jr. and Nelson, J.: Oral antibiotic therapy for skeletal infection of children. II. Therapy of osteomyelitis and suppurative arthritis. Journal of Pediatrics 92: 485 (1978).

Turk, D.C.: A comparison of chloramphenicol and ampicillin as bactericidal agents for *Haemophilus influenzae* type B. Journal of Medical Microbiology 10: 127 (1977).

Warrington, R.J.; Simons, F.E.R.; Ho, H.W.; Gorski, B.A. and Tse, K.S.: Diagnosis of penicillin allergy . by skin testing: The Manitoba experience. Canadian Medical Association Journal 118: 787 (1978).

Yaffe, S.J.; Gerbracht, L.M.; Mosovitch, L.L.; Mattar, M.E.; Danish, M. and Jusko, W.J.: Pharmacokinetics of methicillin in patients with cystic fibrosis. Journal of Infectious Diseases 135: 828 (1977).

Zinner, S.H.; Denny-Brown, B.C.; Braun, P.; Burke, J.P.; Toala, P. and Kass, E.H.: Risk of infection with intravenous indwelling catheters: Effect of application of antibiotic ointment. Journal of Infectious Diseases 120: 616 (1969).

Chapter II

Respiratory Infections

H.C. Spratt, G.A. Ahronheim and M.I. Marks

Respiratory infections are the most frequent clinical problems encountered in acute childhood medicine. In this chapter we will discuss the more common severe bacterial infections of the upper and lower respiratory tracts.

1. Otitis Media

Otitis media of childhood is highly prevalent, and is the subject of much continuing research in pathogenesis, prevention and therapy. The condition has been the subject of several recent reviews (Benjamin and Dorman, 1977; Bluestone and Shurin, 1974; Rowe, 1975).

1.1 Pathogenic Organisms

The predominance of *Streptococcus pneumoniae* (the pneumococcus) and *Haemophilus influenzae* as primary pathogens in otitis media is well recognised (Howard et al., 1974; Howie et al., 1970; Kamme et al., 1971; Schwartz et al., 1977). Staphylococci, other streptococci, and neisseriae may be identified in a minority of cases; *Staphylococcus epidermidis* was identified as the pathogenic agent in 8% of children in one series (Feigin et al., 1973).

The role of Gram-negative enteric bacteria in neonatal otitis media is controversial. One series implicated organisms such as *E. coli* and *Klebsiella pneumoniae* in the majority of cases (Bland, 1972), but two more recent studies indicate that the usual respiratory organisms found in older children also predominate in infants in the first weeks of life (Shurin et al., 1976; Tetzlaff et al., 1977). Anaerobic bacteria have been found in childhood otitis, but their significance is not clear (Brook et al., 1976).

Viruses and mycoplasmata do not appear to play a significant aetiological role in acute otitis, although they may be involved in early pathogenesis (Klein and Teele, 1976).

1.2 Clinical Features and Diagnosis

Infants with acute otitis media usually present with non-specific symptoms of irritability and anorexia, often with accompanying fever. Ear pulling may alert the parents' attention in the absence of other symptoms. Clinical diagnosis relies on abnormalities of the tympanic membrane, including texture, shape, bony landmarks and light reflex (Bluestone and Shurin, 1974; Eavey et al., 1976); impaired mobility of the drum may be obvious on simple pneumatic otoscopy, and can be demonstrated by tympanometry (Bluestone and Shurin, 1974; Shurin et al., 1977). Forceful movement of the drum may be painful. Redness by itself is an unreliable sign, but may justify a second examination.

Tympanocentesis with Gram stain and culture of middle ear fluid provides valuable laboratory confirmation in selected cases (Howard et al., 1976; Howie et al., 1970). Circumstances justifying this procedure include: otitis in the neonate, otitis in patients with abnormal or compromised host defenses, failure of presumably adequate therapy, and suppurative complications such as meningitis. Severe otalgia, unrelieved by analgesics or antibiotics and associated with a bulging tympanic membrane, may be an indication for tympanocentesis or myringotomy (Rowe, 1975).

1.3 Complications

Short term complications of acute otitis media include drum perforation, mastoiditis, meningitis, subdural effusion, and lateral sinus thrombosis with associated intracranial hypertension. Chronic serous otitis media, with conductive hearing loss due to persistent middle ear effusion, is a common sequel, with the potential for compromising language skills if present during the critical periods of speech development in early childhood (Holm and Kunze, 1969).

1.4 Treatment

1.4.1 Acute Otitis Media

Numerous antibiotic regimens have proved effective. For a number of years oral ampicillin has been widely used, but amoxycillin is gaining in popularity among clinicians because of similar efficacy, better absorption and a lower apparent incidence of drug-associated diarrhoea (Howie et al., 1974; Neu, 1974; Wise and Neu, 1974). With equivalent doses, drug concentrations in middle ear effusions may also be significantly higher with amoxycillin than with ampicillin (Klimek et al., 1977).

Either ampicillin (100mg/kg/day in 4 divided oral doses) or amoxycillin (50 to 75mg/kg/day in 3 divided oral doses) for 7 to 10 days is the treatment of choice for children up to 4 to 6 years of age (in whom *H. influenzae* otitis is the most common pathogen). Penicillin V (50 to 100mg/kg/day in 4 divided oral doses) is appropriate for older children, although *H. influenzae* can also be common in this age group (Schwartz et al., 1977), and in view of the uncertainty of the pathogen in any particular area it may therefore be preferable to use ampicillin or amoxycillin in all paediatric age groups. In the presence of proven penicillin hypersensitivity, the combination of erythromycin (50mg/kg/day in 4 doses) plus sulphonamides (as trisulpha-pyrimidines or similar short-acting agents, 120mg/kg/day in 4 doses) is an effective alternative (Howard et al., 1976). Treatment failure may be due to unexpected organisms which may be identified by middle ear aspiration and culture; ampicillin resistant strains of *H. influenzae* have been recognised (Abbott and Faoagali, 1977; Schwartz et al., 1978; Shurin et al., 1976; Syriopoulou et al., 1976) and may respond satisfactorily to erythromycin plus sulphonamides (Khan et al., 1976), obviating the need for a potentially more toxic alternative such as chloramphenicol.

A number of clinical trials have suggested that co-trimoxazole (trimethoprim plus sulphamethoxazole) is also an effective alternative (e.g. Cameron et al., 1975; Quick, 1975). Among the cephalosporins, cephalexin has been found reasonably effective, but its higher relapse rate and greater expense militate against its routine use (McLinn et al., 1975; Stechenberg et al., 1976). Cephalexin should be reserved, along with the semi synthetic antistaphylococcal penicillins, for the uncommon case of recalcitrant otitis media shown to be due to a penicillin resistant staphylococcus.

Adjunctive decongestant therapy is of unproven efficacy in acute otitis media (Rowe, 1975). Except as an aid for cerumenolysis, ear drops of various sorts are of no value (Editorial, 1976).

1.4.2 Recurrent Otitis Media

Recurrent otitis is a common problem in infants, and no definitive therapy is yet available. The cause may be a combination of poor or seemingly inappropriate immunological response (Sloyer et al., 1974, 1975), eustachian tube dysfunction (Bluestone and Beery, 1976), and the wide range of infecting organisms and serotypes. Recent trials of polyvalent pneumococcal vaccines have achieved some reduction in the frequency of otitic attacks in selected cases (Howie et al., 1976). Antimicrobial prophylaxis is another possibility, with sulphafurazole (sulfisoxazole) yielding promising results in one clinical trial (Perrin et al., 1974).

Tympanostomy tubes, with or without adenoidectomy, is a common surgical approach which may provide temporary benefit, but this remains of unproven safety and value (Paradise, 1977; Perrin, 1974).

2. Acute Sinusitis

Inflammatory changes of the mucosa of the paranasal sinuses may be found in infections due to bacteria and viruses and in allergic states. Persistent sinusitis is likely to accompany underlying diseases such as cystic fibrosis, immunodeficiency states, and anatomical abnormalities (Friedberg, 1976).

2.1 Pathogenic Organisms

As in adults (Evans et al., 1975), the most common identifiable pathogens in acute sinusitis are organisms commonly found in the normal nasopharynx, i.e. the pneumococcus, *H. influenzae,* and less frequently β-haemolytic streptococci and *S. aureus.* Positive identification of the pathogen requires its demonstration in uncontaminated material removed directly from the involved sinus, generally by direct sinus puncture or meatal aspiration — procedures rarely performed in children. Therefore, the precise bacterial aetiologies of acute purulent sinusitis remain to be defined in children. In an individual case, Gram stain of a purulent nasal discharge may be useful, but cultures of nasally collected exudates are only modestly helpful.

2.2 Clinical Features and Diagnosis

The most consistent symptoms of sinusitis in children are purulent rhinorrhoea, persistent cough, and associated otitis media (Kogutt and Swischuk, 1973). Other classical clinical features such as nasal obstruction, spontaneous pain, maxillary tenderness, toothache, and abnormal transillumination may be absent in children. Radiological 'clouding' of sinuses may reflect prior infection, mucosal thickening due to nasal allergies, or simple variation in sinus development and aeration.

2.3 Complications

Complications include orbital cellulitis, cavernous sinus thrombosis, frontal or maxillary osteomyelitis, and intracranial extension of infection (Hawkins and Clark, 1977; Kutnick and Kerth, 1976).

2.4 Treatment

Treatment includes the promotion of adequate sinus drainage, topical decongestants, local heat, humidification, analgesics, and antibiotic therapy directed at the
suspected organism (Evans et al., 1975; Kutnick and Kerth, 1976; Quick and Payne,
1972).

Ampicillin (100mg/kg/day) or amoxycillin (75mg/kg/day) are appropriate in
children under 5 years of age. Numerous other antibiotics have also been used with
generally satisfactory results — e.g. penicillin V, co-trimoxazole, cephalosporins, etc.
(Agbim, 1975; Quick, 1975) — suggesting that empirical antibiotic therapy may be
less important than adequate drainage and symptomatic treatment. Nevertheless,
pathogens may be eliminated from infected sinuses and recalcitrant disease may improve when adequate concentrations of the appropriate antibiotic are reached in the
purulent secretions (Axelsson and Brorson, 1973, 1974; Carenfelt et al., 1975; Evans
et al., 1975).

3. Orbital Cellulitis

3.1 Pathogenic Organisms

The most common organisms isolated in children with orbital cellulitis include
S. aureus, H. influenzae, pneumococci and β-haemolytic streptococci, which may be
isolated from cultures of the blood or of neighbouring structures (Haynes and
Cramblett, 1967; Watters et al., 1976). *H. influenzae* cellulitis may occur without an
adjacent focus of infection (Gellady et al., 1977).

3.2 Clinical Features and Diagnosis

Early orbital cellulitis, with erythema and oedema of the eyelids and periorbital
tissues, may progress to involvement of deeper orbital tissues marked by chemosis,
proptosis and ophthalmoplegia. Although sinusitis and ethmoiditis are the most common antecedents (Chandler et al., 1970; Hawkins and Clark, 1977; Haynes and
Cramblett, 1967; Kutnick and Kerth, 1976; Watters et al., 1976), orbital cellulitis
may also be a complication of, and in its early stages difficult to distinguish from,
local processes such as buccal cellulitis, insect bite, trauma, or aggravated conjunctivitis. Fever is often marked, and bacteraemia is frequent (Watters et al., 1976).

Blood cultures are the key to precise diagnosis. Ultrasonography or computerised tomography may delineate orbital abscess formation, a major complication
(Coleman, 1972; Wright et al., 1975).

3.3 Complications

Complications include optic nerve infarction, pan-ophthalmitis, cavernous sinus thrombosis, osteomyelitis of the orbit, and intracranial extension. Prognosis in frank orbital cellulitis depends on the presence or absence of complications and their early recognition and treatment.

3.4 Treatment

Aggressive antibacterial therapy has been associated with a remarkable decrease in morbidity and mortality (Watters et al., 1976). Pending results of bacterial cultures, the combination of ampicillin (200mg/kg/day) and an antistaphylococcal penicillin (e.g. oxacillin or cloxacillin, 150mg/kg/day) is appropriate and should be given intravenously. Chloramphenicol or co-trimoxazole may be used in penicillin hypersensitivity and in infections due to ampicillin resistant *H. influenzae*. Penicillin G (100,000u/kg/day IV) may be used alone in cases shown to be caused by pneumococci or streptococci.

In addition to appropriate antibiotic therapy, cases of frank orbital cellulitis require careful surgical and radiological evaluation, with early drainage of any demonstrated orbital abscess, infected sinus or dental abscess (Kutnick and Kerth, 1976).

4. Pharyngitis and Tonsillitis

4.1 Pathogenic Organisms

The great majority of throat infections are non-bacterial in aetiology. The group A β-haemolytic streptococcus is the most important bacterial pathogen (primarily because of its high incidence and its association with late non-suppurative complications such as rheumatic fever) and in general, is the only bacterial pathogen to be sought. *Corynebacterium diphtheriae* and *Neisseria gonorrhoeae* (van Overbeek, 1976) are also significant pathogens. *Pseudomonas aeruginosa* and *Candida albicans* may be important in immunocompromised patients.

4.2 Complications

The high prevalence in former years of rheumatic fever, scarlet fever and acute glomerulonephritis in association with tonsillitis, led to exhaustive epidemiological studies of β-haemolytic streptococcal carriage and disease. Qualitative streptococcal screening of ill children and contacts continues to be employed in many centres (Zimmerman et al., 1974).

The discovery of a very high throat carriage rate amongst asymptomatic children (Quinn et al., 1957; Zanen et al., 1959) has led to much work with semi-quantitative culture methods to distinguish carriage from disease, the applicability of which remains to be proven (Bell and Smith, 1976; Breese et al., 1970; Ross, 1971). Serological methods have also been applied to distinguish carriage from disease: in one study, using a combination of culture and streptococcal antibody techniques, a low yield ($<$ 20%) of probable streptococcal disease was found amongst children presenting with uncomplicated pharyngitis (Kaplan et al., 1971).

4.3 Treatment

Conflicting data, and a reduction in the incidence of non-suppurative sequelae of streptococcal infection in developing countries (Quinn and Federspiel, 1974) make it difficult to recommend guidelines for the management of individual cases and practice policy. Using simple culture methods, the isolation of a group A β-haemolytic streptococcus should be considered significant if associated with clinical disease. The treatment of choice remains penicillin. Oral penicillin G or V must be administered for 7 to 10 days to significantly decrease the likelihood of non-suppurative complications (Markowitz and Gordis, 1972). Failure of therapy is frequently associated with poor compliance, and unless patient education and follow-up are optimal, intramuscular benzathine penicillin G may be more satisfactory. A single injection of 300,000 to 600,000 units in children will eliminate the streptococcus in 95% of patients (Chamovitz et al., 1954). Relapses may be associated with streptococcal carriage in household contacts, which may be dealt with by simultaneous culturing and antibiotic therapy.

Oral erythromycin is appropriate in cases of proven penicillin hypersensitivity (Derrick and Dillon, 1976); however, the use of other antibiotics for uncomplicated pharyngitis is rarely indicated and should be avoided if possible.

5. Epiglottitis

Epiglottitis is an uncommon but serious and potentially lethal disease and is a true paediatric emergency (Berenberg and Kevy, 1958).

5.1 Pathogenic Organisms

Haemophilus influenzae type b accounts for more than 95% of childhood cases of epiglottitis (Branefors-Helander and Jeppsson, 1975; Margolis et al., 1975). Blood cultures are positive in over 90 % of cases presenting without prior antibiotic therapy. The age incidence of epiglottitis is less restricted than for other forms of *H. influenzae* infections, and cases in adolescents and adults are well documented (Baxter, 1967; Branefors-Helander and Jeppsson, 1975; Robins and Fitz-Hugh, 1971).

5.2 Clinical Features and Diagnosis

Clinical features include a short febrile prodrome followed by intense sore throat, dysphagia, drooling, stridor, neck extension, dyspnoea and toxicity, with rapid progression to airway obstruction (Bass et al., 1974). Diagnosis is suspected by the history and may be confirmed by direct visualisation. However, direct inspection of the pharynx is dangerous, as simple manipulation such as the use of a tongue depressor may precipitate airway occlusion.

A lateral radiograph of the soft tissues of the neck may show a swollen and deformed epiglottis (Dunbar, 1961); when available without delay, this study is of diagnostic value.

No case of suspected epiglottitis should be managed without preparation for an immediate intubation or tracheostomy while evaluation and treatment are underway (Johnson et al., 1974). Differential diagnosis includes subglottic croup, inhaled foreign body, and rarely, measles and diphtheria.

5.3 Complications

Respiratory complications such as pneumothorax, pneumomediastinum, or late laryngeal stricture more commonly follow tracheostomy, and are infrequent. Other complications including otitis media, cervical lymphadenitis, pneumonitis, meningitis or septic arthritis may be seen in up to a third of cases (Branefors-Helander and Jeppsson, 1975; Molteni, 1976).

5.4 Treatment

Several centres have reported their experience with an expectant policy of careful management without early intubation or tracheostomy (Bass et al., 1974; Rapkin, 1973; Strome and Jaffe, 1974). However, because of the unpredictability of abrupt respiratory arrest and the cumulative problems of resuscitation, this policy cannot be routinely recommended. It may be justified in the minority of cases without respiratory distress when strict monitoring is assured, but otherwise nasotracheal intubation is recommended for all confirmed cases.

Attention to supportive care, pulmonary toilet and antibacterial therapy contribute to reduced morbidity (Battaglia and Lockhart, 1975; Geraci, 1968; Weber et al., 1976). The clinical emergency responds promptly to intubation, suction and oxygenation. Intensive nursing care is required, as accidental extubation or tube obstruction may be fatal. Clinical toxicity often subsides within 48 hours of starting antibiotic therapy, and the nasotracheal tube can usually be safely removed within 3 days (Battaglia and Lockhart, 1975; Geraci, 1968; Weber et al., 1976).

Intravenous ampicillin (200mg/kg/day) is recommended for antibiotic therapy. Although ampicillin resistant strains of *H. influenzae* are being recognised with increasing frequency, to date it appears that ampicillin alone, with adequate supportive care and airway assurance, is appropriate initial therapy, presumably due to high serum and local concentrations of the drug. Chloramphenicol (50mg/kg/day IV) is an appropriate alternative, especially in the presence of known penicillin hypersensitivity. However, chloramphenicol resistance has also been described recently in clinical isolates of *H. influenzae* (Center for Disease Control, 1976), and a search for other effective agents is actively under way (Marks, 1975; McGowan et al., 1976; Smith, 1976).

The adjunctive use of corticosteroids has been proposed for acute management (Strome and Jaffe, 1974); however, because of the pathogenetic mechanisms apparently involved — bacterial invasion and polymorphonuclear leucocyte exudation — and the lack of clearcut benefits, such therapy does not appear justified.

6. Pertussis

Pertussis remains a controversial subject; the aetiological role of viruses in the syndrome (Baraff, 1978; Connor, 1970), virus-*Bordetella pertussis* interplay (Nelson et al., 1975), and the risk/benefit analysis of vaccine programmes (Miller et al., 1974; Preston, 1976; Preston and Stanbridge, 1975) are among the many contentious issues (Linnemann et al., 1974; Wilkins and Bass, 1976).

6.1 Pathogenic Organisms

The pertussis syndrome is most commonly caused by *Bordetella pertussis* and, rarely, by *B. parapertussis, B. bronchiseptica* and respiratory viruses. A recent prospective study (Baraff et al., 1978) gives strong support to the view that pertussis is caused by *B. pertussis* in the large majority of cases, and that adenoviruses seldom play a direct aetiological role. The data also showed diminished recovery of the organism in immunised children compared with non-immunised children, inferring the presence of local immunity in vaccine recipients.

A preliminary study of the pathogenesis of pertussis has described physiological responses compatible with β_2-adrenoceptor blockade in the liver and the bronchial tree (Badr-El-Din et al., 1976b): these changes were reversed by the administration of the β_2-adrenergic stimulant, salbutamol (Badr-El-Din et al., 1976a). Further studies of this approach in human disease seem warranted.

6.2 Clinical Features and Diagnosis

The classic three-phase clinical course of pertussis is well recognised: non-specific upper respiratory symptoms, followed by a period of severe and characteristic paroxysmal cough, and protracted convalescence. Diagnosis is strengthened by a positive contact history, the absence of fever, and a peripheral lymphocytosis. Confirmation relies on identification of *B. pertussis* from nasopharyngeal swabs, generally by isolation on Bordet-Gengou agar or by visualisation with fluorescent antibody. Late presentation, and the fastidious nature of the organism, may contribute to the low yield of *B. pertussis* isolates in many centres (Bass et al., 1975).

6.3 Complications

Complications of pertussis include pneumonia, atelectasis, otitis and infrequently, encephalopathy. Post-pertussis bronchiectasis has become uncommon in recent years.

6.4 Treatment

Supportive care — gentle physiotherapy, airway suction, and humidified air — is the mainstay of therapy, with antibiotics playing at best a minor role. Erythromycin reduces communicability but does not lessen symptoms (Bass et al., 1969; Wilkins and Bass, 1976). Symptomatic contacts in the pre-paroxysmal phase may be protected from severe disease by erythromycin (Linnemann et al., 1975; Wilkins and Bass, 1976), which offers rational prophylaxis for exposed non-immune infants. The recommended dose of erythromycin is 50mg/kg/day for 10 to 14 days. Hyperimmune serotherapy is not effective (Balagtas et al., 1971).

6.5 Role of Immunisation

Vaccine protection is reliable (Noah, 1976; Preston, 1976) and recommended (Stuart-Harris, 1975). Young infants are apparently not protected by maternal antibodies and if exposed are at risk of severe disease. Life threatening whooping cough is usually confined to children under two years of age.

Scepticism about the value of pertussis vaccine is unwarranted. Although adverse effects of immunisation are bothersome, our experience with the vaccine and with illness in unimmunised children lead to this opinion.

7. Pneumonia

Pneumonia constitutes less than 5% of acute respiratory disease in children, with non-bacterial causes predominating (Foy et al., 1973; Glezen and Denny, 1973; Zollar et al., 1973). Specific viral agents are often associated with well defined lower respiratory syndromes other than pneumonia, e.g. respiratory syncytial virus with bronchiolitis, parainfluenza viruses with tracheobronchitis (croup), etc. [Glezen and Denny, 1973].

7.1 Pathogenic Organisms

The most common bacterial pathogens recognised as causes of spontaneous pneumonia include the pneumococcus, *Staphylococcus aureus,* and *Haemophilus influenzae* (Honig et al., 1973; Potter and Fischer, 1977). Pneumonia due to Gram-negative enteric bacilli occurs predominantly in newborn infants and in children with compromised defences. The group B streptococcus *(Strep. agalactiae)* causes a fulminating pneumonia early in the neonatal period which is difficult to distinguish from hyaline membrane disease (Ablow et al., 1976; Hemming et al., 1976; Vollman et al., 1976). Staphylococcal pneumonia is most common in infants, and following viral pneumonia (measles and influenza).

Mycoplasma pneumoniae may be the most common cause in school aged children and young adults (Denny et al., 1971; Fernald et al., 1975; Foy et al., 1973; Glezen and Denny, 1973). *Chlamydia trachomatis* has recently been associated with a distinctive indolent pneumonia in young infants (Beem and Saxon, 1977a; Harrison et al., 1978). Primary tuberculosis must also not be forgotten.

7.2 Clinical Features and Diagnosis

Except for classic lobar pneumonia in the older child which is usually pneumococcal, and group B streptococcal neonatal pneumonia, there are no clear-cut pneumonitic syndromes pathognomonic of any specific bacterial agent. The patient's age, relevant history, and epidemiology usually provide as much useful information as the clinical examination, with laboratory data such as peripheral leucocytosis (Shuttleworth and Charney, 1971) and the demonstration of abundant pus cells in sputum helping to substantiate an impression of bacterial pneumonia. An elevated acute cold-agglutinin titre in a school aged child with pneumonia strongly suggests *Mycoplasma pneumoniae* infection (Denny et al., 1971).

The microscopic and culture examination of expectorated sputum, of borderline value in adults (Barrett-Connor, 1971), is often unhelpful in paediatrics because of the difficulty in obtaining a satisfactory specimen. Transtracheal aspiration is impractical in infants and children and bronchoscopy (Bartlett et al., 1976) and laryngoscopic aspiration do not obviate the risk of contamination by pharyngeal flora. Carefully collected and inspected specimens may reveal small bronchial plugs or purulent mucus which, when the stained smear contains abundant polymorphonuclear leucocytes and no squamous epithelial cells, may be bacteriologically useful (Murray and Washington, 1975).

Nevertheless, a definitive diagnosis depends on isolation of a pathogen from blood, pleural fluid or lung. Direct percutaneous lung puncture, with smear and culture of the aspirate, is usually a benign procedure, and is justified in selected cases (Davidson et al., 1976; Mimica et al., 1971). In complex cases such as patients with cancer or on immunosuppressive therapy, open lung biopsy may be required to distinguish treatable infectious causes of pulmonary disease — i.e. bacterial pneumonia, *Pneumocystitis carinii* infection, etc. — from neoplasm, fibrosis, or chemotherapy toxicity (Mason et al., 1977; Wolff et al., 1977).

Mycoplasma may be isolated by direct inoculation of throat washings or sputum on mycoplasma media, and infection may be documented serologically.

7.3 Complications

Spontaneously occurring pneumonia is often a bacteraemic illness, possibly leading to extrapulmonary foci of infection. Local complications may include lung abscess, empyema, pneumothorax and atelectasis, while haematogenous spread may lead to distant complications such as meningitis.

Deaths from promptly diagnosed and properly treated pneumonia in the otherwise healthy patient are happily now rare. Prognosis for survivors is excellent. Pulmonary function in long term follow-up of childhood pneumonitis generally returns to normal (Ceruti et al., 1971; Wise et al., 1966).

7.4 Treatment

Antibiotic therapy is often empirical in the absence of good bacteriology. The choice may be guided by epidemiological considerations, such as those summarised above, remembering that most paediatric pneumonia in otherwise healthy children is non-bacterial.

7.4.1 Pneumococcal Pneumonia

Pneumococcal pneumonia is managed with parenteral penicillin G (25,000 to 100,000u/kg/day); recent studies in adults indicate that massive dosage is unnecessary in the uncomplicated case (Brewin et al., 1974) and this may be expected to be applicable to children as well. As toxicity abates, oral therapy is appropriate; penicillin V (25 to 50mg/kg/day) is given until clinical signs have resolved and recovery is evident. The usual total course of antibiotic therapy averages one to two weeks. In penicillin hypersensitive patients, a cephalosporin such as cephalothin (100mg/kg/day IV) or cephalexin (50mg/kg/day orally) may be used. Sensitivity tests should be performed if the response to therapy is poor and if erythromycin (50mg/kg/day) is used.

Uncomplicated pneumonia due to other streptococci (not enterococci) is managed similarly.

7.4.2 Staphylococcal Pneumonia

Staphylococcal pneumonia must initially be managed with parenteral semi-synthetic antistaphylococcal penicillins such as cloxacillin or oxacillin (100 to 150mg/kg/day); a cephalosporin such as cephalothin (100mg/kg/day IV) is an acceptable alternative in penicillin hypersensitive patients. Penicillin may be substituted only after demonstration of the organism's susceptibility.

To forestall relapse and suppurative complications such as abscess or empyema, at least 3 weeks antibiotic therapy should be given. When fever, toxicity and acute illness have abated, well absorbed agents such as cloxacillin or dicloxacillin may be substituted by the oral route if adequate bacterial activity can be demonstrated in the serum.

7.4.3 *H. influenzae* Pneumonia

H. influenzae, as discussed in the section on epiglottitis (section 5.4), is treated with either ampicillin or chloramphenicol; co-trimoxazole may also be given as an alternative. Cephalosporins are generally less potent *in vitro* and have not yet been shown to be clinically effective against *H. influenzae*.

7.4.4 Neonatal Pneumonia

Neonates, in whom Gram-negative enteric bacterial and group B streptococcal pneumonias are frequent, are treated initially with the combination of an aminoglycoside (e.g. kanamycin or gentamicin) and a penicillin. Therapy is subsequently modified if necessary on the basis of culture and susceptibility results. Recent *in vitro* and animal studies suggest that group B streptococci, despite good susceptibility to

Table I. Guide to the use of antibacterial drugs in paediatric respiratory infections

Antibacterial drug	Dose and route	Side Effects
Amoxycillin	50 to 75mg/kg/day po divided q8h	As for ampicillin, with lower incidence of dose-related side effects (e.g. diarrhoea)
Ampicillin	200mg/kg/day IV divided q6h 100mg/kg/day po divided q6h	Diarrhoea, rash, fever and superinfections. Rarely, haemolytic anaemia, interstitial nephritis, colitis syndrome NB Maculopapular rash is not a contraindication to continuing therapy, or use of a penicillin subsequently. True urticaria is a hypersensitivity reaction, which generally contraindicates further use
Cephalothin	75 to 150mg/kg/day IV divided q6h	Hypersensitivity reactions, fever, rash, blood dyscrasia, liver enzyme elevation, nephritis Painful IM
Chloramphenicol	100mg/kg/day (as succinate) IV divided q6h 100mg/kg/day po divided q6h NB 25mg/kg/day up to 2 weeks of age, then 50mg/kg/day in 1 dose. Serum levels should be monitored.	Bone marrow depression, vasomotor collapse in the newborn (dose-related), haemolysis in G6PD deficiency, gastrointestinal symptoms, superinfections Should not be given IM
Cloxacillin	100 to 150mg/kg/day IV divided q6h 50 to 100mg/kg/day po divided q6h	Similar to other penicillins
Co-trimoxazole (trimethoprim + sulphamethoxazole in a 1:5 ratio)	15 to 30mg sulphamethoxazole/kg/day IV divided q12h 25 to 50mg sulphamethoxazole/kg/day po divided q12h	As for sulphonamides
Dicloxacillin	50 to 100mg/kg/day po divided q6h	Similar to other penicillins
Erythromycin	30 to 50mg/kg/day po divided q6h 40 to 70mg/kg/day IV divided q6h (slow infusion)	Gastrointestinal disturbances, fever, rash, superinfections. Estolate may cause reversible intrahepatic cholestasis (if given for more than 10 to 14 days)

Drug	Dosage	Notes
Ethambutol	15mg/kg/day po once daily	Retrobulbar neuritis at higher dose levels, hypersensitivity reactions (limited experience in children)
Gentamicin	*Infants less than 2kg:* 5mg/kg/day IV divided q12 to 24h for first week, then 7.5mg/kg/day divided q12h *Infants more than 2kg:* 5 to 7.5mg/kg/day IV divided q12h for first week, then q8h *Older children:* 5 to 6mg/kg/day IV divided q8h	Ototoxic and possibly nephrotoxic Dosages up to 7.5mg/kg/day may be used for short periods for severe infections Ototoxicity may depend on peak blood levels
Isoniazid	*Therapy:* Oral: 15 to 20mg/kg/day divided q12h (up to a maximum of 600mg daily): IM: 10mg/kg/day divided q12h *Prophylaxis:* 10mg/kg/day (up to 300mg daily)	Gastrointestinal disturbances, rashes (may be acneiform), haemolysis in G6PD deficiency Neurotoxicity and hepatotoxicity are rare in children
Kanamycin	*Infants less than 2kg:* 15mg/kg/day IV divided q12h for first week, then 20mg/kg/day divided q12h *Infants more than 2kg:* 20mg/kg/day IV divided q12h for first week, then 30mg/kg/day divided q8h *Older children:* 15mg/kg/day IV divided q12h	Ototoxic Potential for neuromuscular blockade following rapid infusion (administer slowly over 30 to 60 minutes) May aggravate pre-existing renal disease
Para-aminosalicylic acid (PAS)	250 to 300mg/kg/day po divided q6h	Gastrointestinal disturbances, hypersensitivity reactions, thrombocytopenia, haemolysis in G6PD deficiency
Penicillin G	25,000 to 100,000u/kg/day IV divided q6h; po: 1hr before or 2hrs after meals	Shares same spectrum of side effects as ampicillin, with generally lower incidence
Penicillin V	25 to 50mg/kg/day po divided q6h	
Penicillin G benzathine	300,000 to 1,200,000u IM (single dose)	
Rifampicin	15 to 20mg/kg/day po once daily (up to a maximum of 600mg)	Bone marrow depression; hepatotoxicity and nephrotoxicity are uncommon and usually reversible Avoid intermittent dosage
Sulphonamides Sulphadiazine Triple sulpha Sulphafurazole Sulphamethoxazole	120mg/kg/day IV divided q6h 120 to 150mg/kg/day po divided q6h 25 to 50mg/kg/day po divided q6h	Gastrointestinal disturbances, crystalluria (alkalinise urine), hypersensitivity reactions, haemolysis in G6PD deficiency, bone marrow suppression, kernicterus in the newborn

penicillin by the usual techniques, are killed more rapidly with such a combination than by penicillins alone (Deveikis et al., 1977; Schauf et al., 1976); however, clinical correlations are not yet available. Uncomplicated neonatal pneumonia due to these organisms is usually treated for at least two weeks.

7.4.5 Mycoplasmal Pneumonia

The efficacy of antibiotic therapy in mycoplasmal pneumonitis has been a controversial subject. Erythromycin (50mg/kg/day orally) and tetracyclines appear to decrease, with similar efficacy, the duration of fever and pulmonary infiltrates, although a dramatic improvement (such as that with penicillin against pneumococci) is not seen (Denny et al., 1971). Tetracyclines should however, be avoided in children under 8 years of age because of various hazards such as dental staining (American Academy of Pediatrics, 1975; Grossman et al., 1971).

Clindamycin appeared to be ineffective in a controlled clinical trial (Smilack et al., 1974).

7.4.6 Chlamydial Pneumonia

A preliminary report has suggested that sulphonamides or erythromycin may be useful in chlamydial pneumonia in infants (Beem and Saxon, 1977b), but controlled studies are not yet available.

8. Pleural Empyema

Epidemiological studies of (non-tuberculous) empyema associated with pneumonia in children have shown a sharp decline in incidence, morbidity and mortality (Bechamps et al., 1970; Ravitch and Fein, 1961), attributable in great measure to antibiotics and improved management.

8.1 Pathogenic Organisms

Empyema classically was a consequence of pneumococcal pneumonia, but in the antibiotic era, *S. aureus* has become the most common cause in children (Bechamps et al., 1970; Cattaneo and Kilman, 1973); other bacteria such as streptococci and Gram-negative bacilli are also encountered, but *H. influenzae* has been surprisingly infrequently described (Riley and Bracken, 1965). Pleural effusions have been recognised to occur with mycoplasmal, viral, and rickettsial pneumonias (Caughey, 1977;

Fine et al., 1970; Grix and Giammona, 1974). Cystic fibrosis may present in infancy with staphylococcal pneumonia and empyema, and appropriate testing is recommended in all such infants (Taussig et al., 1974).

8.2 Clinical Features and Diagnosis

Acute untreated empyema is usually accompanied by marked toxicity and symptoms and signs of pneumonia with effusion. Partially treated or chronic cases may have an insidious presentation.

Following radiographic demonstration of a probably infectious pleural effusion, investigations should include diagnostic thoracentesis with cytological, biochemical and microbiological studies (Carr, 1973). Immediately prior to actual thoracentesis, the puncture site should be aseptically prepared and a swab culture taken to monitor efficacy and possible contamination of the aspirate; a blood culture should follow the procedure. Pleural biopsy is indicated in suspected tuberculous effusion, and an acid-fast as well as a Gram stain should be performed on a smear of the fluid. Selection of culture media may be critical, not only for recovery of mycobacteria (Lowenstein-Jensen agar) or *Haemophilus* spp. (chocolate, Levinthal or Fildes agar), but also, in the event of prior antibiotic therapy, of cell-wall-defective bacteria ('L-forms') for which hypertonic media may be useful (Irwin et al., 1975).

8.3 Treatment

Therapy for empyema consists of surgical drainage and aggressive antibiotic therapy based on culture and sensitivity studies. A parenteral semisynthetic anti-staphylococcal penicillin such as cloxacillin or nafcillin (100mg/kg/day IV) is recommended for initial therapy in children pending identification of a pathogen, because of the preponderance of *S. aureus*. In otherwise uncomplicated staphylococcal empyema, following resolution of fever, evidence of sterilisation of the pleural space, and resolution of the effusion, a well absorbed drug of this class — e.g. cloxacillin or dicloxacillin — may be continued orally for an additional 1 to 2 weeks at a dose of 75 to 100mg/kg/day (monitored if necessary by serum bactericidal studies against the patient's organism); this permits greater mobility and eliminates the risks of thrombophlebitis and the pain of multiple venipunctures for the convalescent patient. The prolonged duration of therapy may also reduce the risk of relapse, although controlled studies are lacking on this point.

Other antibiotics may be used as indicated by the initial Gram stain and subsequent culture results: penicillin G (100,000u/kg/day IV) is appropriate for pneumococci and non-enterococcal streptococci, penicillin sensitive staphylococci, and most anaerobes (other than *Bacteroides fragilis,* for which chloramphenicol

[100mg/kg/day IV or orally] or clindamycin [25 to 50mg/kg/day IV] is recommended). *H. influenzae* is treated with ampicillin (150 to 200mg/kg/day IV) or, if β-lactamase-producing, with co-trimoxazole or chloramphenicol. Enteric Gram-negative bacilli may require aminoglycoside treatment (e.g. kanamycin, 15 to 20mg/kg/day, or gentamicin, 5 to 7.5mg/kg/day).

Closed tube thoracostomy is recommended for initial management of empyema, and its importance cannot be overemphasised (Bechamps et al., 1970; Cattaneo and Kilman, 1973; van de Water, 1970). Frequent thoracentesis has been advocated for infants (Bechamps et al., 1970) but rapid drainage may be achieved by the non-operative percutaneous insertion of a polyethylene tube until the infant is sufficiently stable for operative intervention to be considered. Chest physiotherapy is also an important additional part of therapy.

With proper management, the prognosis of childhood bacterial empyema is good (Cattaneo and Kilman, 1973; Wise et al., 1966) and fibrothorax has become rare.

9. Croup, Bronchiolitis and Bronchitis

9.1 Pathogenic Organisms

Croup and bronchiolitis are specific paediatric syndromes, and in anatomical terms, could be considered equivalent to acute bronchitis of adults. The work of Parrott et al. (1962) firmly established their viral causation in children, although an association with *H. influenzae* may rarely exist with croup. Classical croup in the form of laryngeal diphtheria is now very rare.

Acute bronchitis is usually manifested by persistent cough; low grade fever may also be present. Influenza, parainfluenza, and adenoviruses are the usual aetiological agents. Secondary bacterial infections due to *Str. pneumoniae* or *H. influenzae* may occur in viral or asthmatic bronchitis. Primary bacterial bronchitis in pertussis, mycoplasma infection or tuberculosis are discussed under these headings (sections 6, 7.4.5, and 10).

9.2 Treatment

Management is based on the relief of airway obstruction and hypoxaemia, with appropriate supportive measures and observation for signs of secondary infection. The rational use of antibiotics is confined to cases of suspected secondary bacterial infection or equivocal periglottic obstruction. Unless the blood culture is positive or x-ray evidence of pneumonia is present, this decision usually depends on the clinical impression, temperature, time course, white clood cell count, sputum microscopy and bacteriology, etc. When antibiotic therapy is thought necessary, ampicillin (100mg/kg/day) or amoxycillin (50mg/kg/day) are recommended with careful observation of the clinical, cytological (sputum) and bacteriological response. Patients with immune deficiencies, bronchiectasis or cystic fibrosis suffer frequent and complicated bacterial bronchitis. Specific antibiotic therapy depends on careful sequential study of the sputum cytology and bacteriology as well as the clinical course (Landau, 1978).

10. Pulmonary Tuberculosis

A comprehensive review of childhood tuberculosis (TB) is beyond the scope of this book and can be found elsewhere (Kendig, 1972; Lincoln and Sewell, 1977). Important recent developments in pulmonary TB include the introduction of rifampicin and the prospect of short duration chemotherapy (Johnston and Wildrick, 1974). Published reports in these areas have primarily been concerned with adults, with relatively little data directly applicable to children.

10.1 Diagnostic Considerations

Tuberculin skin testing (Sewell et al., 1974) has an important role in patient diagnosis and in screening programmes. Multiple puncture tests such as the Tine are reliable for routine use and screening provided any positive reaction is followed up by standardised Mantoux testing. Following intradermal injection of 5 TU (intermediate strength) of Tween-stabilised tuberculin (PPD-S), induration $\geqslant$ 10mm constitutes a positive reaction and necessitates careful evaluation of the patient and family contacts (Sewell et al., 1974). Contact with atypical mycobacteria may give less strong or doubtful reactions.

Mantoux test interpretations may be complicated by prior BCG vaccination (Editorial, 1969). Available data suggest that infants vaccinated at birth tend to be tuberculin-negative a year later, but that reactivity is retained for much longer in children vaccinated at age 6 years (Joncas et al., 1975); however, Mantoux test induration in vaccinees rarely exceeds 20mm, so that any greater reaction makes evaluation for tuberculous infection mandatory. Tuberculin testing is not invalidated by the simultaneous administration of live viral vaccines (Brickman et al., 1975). Tuberculin reactors without demonstrable disease, and small children in close contact with infectious excretors of tubercle bacilli, should receive a one year course of isoniazid (10mg/kg/day; maximum 300mg/day in children) to prevent later development of active TB (American Thoracic Society, 1977; Ferebee, 1970; Hsu, 1974); family contacts should also be screened thoroughly.

Table II. Summary of the treatment of common bacterial respiratory infections of infancy and childhood

---

1. *Acute otitis media*
   a) Either amoxycillin (50 to 75mg/kg/day) or ampicillin (100mg/kg/day) orally for 7 to 10 days is treatment of choice
   b) In penicillin hypersensitive patients, erythromycin (50mg/kg/day) + short acting sulphonamide (120mg/kg/day), or co-trimoxazole
   c) Analgesics for pain
   d) Tympanocentesis for complicated cases and therapeutic failures

2. *Acute sinusitis*
   a) Promote adequate sinus drainage
   b) Symptomatic treatment (e.g. topical decongestants, local heat, humidification, analgesics)
   c) Antibiotic therapy directed at suspected organism (e.g. amoxycillin or ampicillin, co-trimoxazole)

3. *Orbital cellulitis*
   a) Parenteral ampicillin (200mg/kg/day) + antistaphylococcal penicillin (e.g. oxacillin or cloxacillin, 150mg/kg/day) IV, pending results of bacterial cultures
   b) Penicillin G (100,000u/kg/day IV) if due to pneumococci or streptococci
   c) Early drainage of any orbital abscess, infected sinus or dental abscess

4. *Pharyngitis and tonsillitis*
   a) Oral penicillin G or V for 7 to 10 days
   b) Benzathine penicillin (300,000 to 600,000u IM single injection) if compliance suspect
   c) Erythromycin in penicillin hypersensitive patients

5. *Epiglottitis* (NB. a paediatric emergency)
   a) Nasotracheal intubation
   b) Supportive care (incl. airway suction, oxygenation)
   c) Antibiotic therapy — ampicillin (200mg/kg/day IV); chloramphenicol (50mg/kg/day IV) if penicillin hypersensitive

6. *Pertussis*
   a) Supportive care (gentle physiotherapy, airway suction, humidified air)
   b) Erythromycin (50mg/kg/day) for 10 to 14 days to reduce communicability; may also protect symptomatic contacts in pre-paroxysmal phase and exposed non-immunes
   c) Vaccine protection reliable and recommended

7. *Pneumonia*
   a) *Pneumococcal pneumonia:* If toxic, penicillin G (25,000 to 100,000u/kg/day IV) until toxicity abates, followed by oral penicillin V (25 to 50mg/kg/day) until resolution. Use cephalosporins in penicillin hypersensitivity
   b) *Staphylococcal pneumonia:* Antistaphylococcal penicillins (e.g. oxacillin or cloxacillin, 100 to 150mg/kg/day) parenterally until toxicity abates, followed by oral cloxacillin or dicloxacillin (50 to 100mg/kg/day) for at least 3 weeks. Use cephalosporins in penicillin hypersensitivity
   c) *H. influenzae pneumonia:* Treat with ampicillin (200mg/kg/day IV) or chloramphenicol (50mg/kg/ day IV)
   d) *Neonatal pneumonia:* Treat initially with aminoglycoside (e.g. gentamicin or kanamycin) + ampicillin; modify therapy on basis of culture results
   e) *Mycoplasmal pneumonia:* Treat with erythromycin (50mg/kg/day po)

8. *Pleural empyema*
   a) Surgical drainage
   b) Parenteral antistaphylococcal penicillin (e.g. cloxacillin, 100mg/kg/day IV) until resolution, followed by oral cloxacillin or dicloxacillin (75 to 100mg/kg/day) for additional 1 to 2 weeks
   c) Other antibiotics can be substituted as indicated by culture results
   d) Chest physiotherapy

9. *Acute bronchitis*
   a) Treatment essentially symptomatic (e.g. adequate hydration, physiotherapy)
   b) Antibiotics rarely indicated — amoxycillin or ampicillin are drugs of choice; penicillin or a cephalosporin may be used for pneumococcal infection and co-trimoxazole for *H. influenzae*

10.2 Treatment

10.2.1 Isoniazid

Isoniazid (INH) is the mainstay of nearly all anti-TB regimens (American Thoracic Society, 1977; Hsu, 1974; Johnston and Wildrick, 1974). In uncomplicated pulmonary TB, children are given isoniazid at a dosage of 10mg/kg/day up to a maximum of 300mg/day (under age 2 months a reduced dose of 3 to 5mg/kg/day is used); for disseminated or severe disease, 15 to 20mg/kg/day up to a maximum of 450mg/day may be required. Pyridoxine (25 or 50mg/day) may be given to adolescents, as in adults, to prevent the peripheral neuritis which may occur as a side effect of long term isoniazid.

Because of the risk of emergence of mycobacterial resistance during therapy, and increasingly because of the recognition of primary drug resistant strains of *Mycobacterium tuberculosis*, isoniazid should not be used alone. Para-aminosalicylic acid (PAS; 150mg/kg/day) is an important second drug, but is problematical because of gastrointestinal side effects and the frequent difficulty in administering large numbers of tablets to children.

10.2.2 Streptomycin

Streptomycin remains an important drug for initial treatment in disseminated disease or meningitis, or when primary drug resistant strains are a possibility. It is administered intramuscularly in doses of 20 to 40mg/kg (maximum 1.0g/dose) once daily for the first 1 to 3 weeks of therapy, and may be continued thereafter for up to six months when given 2 or 3 times per week, in combination with at least one other drug.

10.2.3 Ethambutol

Ethambutol is widely used in adults but has not gained general acceptance in paediatric anti-TB therapy because of the difficulty in monitoring visual toxicity. When necessary, it has been used in adolescents in doses of 15 to 20mg/kg/day or 50mg/kg twice weekly (Doster et al., 1973).

10.2.4 Rifampicin

The role of rifampicin in childhood pulmonary TB is unclear (Johnston and Wildrick, 1975; Newman et al., 1975), although it appears to be a very useful addition to the treatment of tuberculous meningitis. Although few paediatric studies have been published (Dieu et al., 1970; Gerbeaux et al., 1975; Simon, 1975), and a variety of side effects and toxic manifestations have been recognised (Girling, 1977), the use of rifampicin in the initial treatment of childhood TB is increasing. The paediatric dose of rifampicin is 15mg/kg once daily in the fasting state, infants under one week of age being given no more than 10mg/kg/day.

Intermittent administration of rifampicin is associated with a flu-like syndrome, and should be avoided (Girling, 1977). As with other antituberculosis agents, rifampicin should not be used alone because of the possibility of emerging drug resistance.

10.2.5 Duration of Therapy

Short duration chemotherapy trials of 6, 9 and 12 months in adults have yielded promising results (Addington et al., 1977; British Thoracic and Tuberculosis Association, 1975, 1976; Johnston and Wildrick, 1974; Pilheu, 1977), and are needed in childhood TB; in the meantime, we continue to recommend no less than 12 months (preferably 18) of chemotherapy with two drugs to which the patient's organism is sensitive.

10.2.6 Period of Infectivity

Infectivity is related to airborne transmission and close contact of susceptibles, and in adults falls dramatically once adequate chemotherapy is underway (Bates and Stead, 1974; Gunnels et al., 1974). Current recommendations for adults (in whom hospitalisation is not otherwise required) permit a return to employment when chemotherapy has induced a significant decrease in the number of acid-fast bacilli in sputum, when cough is absent, and when contact with susceptibles in a closed environment is not anticipated (American Thoracic Society, 1973). Although children with primary (non-cavitary) pulmonary TB excrete remarkably few tubercle bacilli and therefore are probably minimally infectious even before treatment, guidelines for the return of a child to school are not well established. The practice in this institution is to keep hospitalisation as brief as possible and, in non-cavitary TB, to permit return to school when cough is resolved. Further studies are needed to prove the apparent safety of this policy.

References

Abbott, G.D. and Faoagali, J.L.: H. influenzae type 6 resistant to ampicillin. New Zealand Medical Journal 86: 301 (1977).

Ablow, R.C.; Driscoll, S.G.; Effman, E.L.; Gross, I.; Jolles, C.J.; Uauy, R. and Warshaw, J.D.: A comparison of early-onset group B streptococcal neonatal infection and the respiratory-distress syndrome of the newborn. New England Journal of Medicine 294: 65-70 (1976).

Addington, W.W.; Agarwal, M.K. and Banner, A.S.: Toward shorter-course antituberculosis chemotherapy. Chest 71: 565 (1977).

Agbim, O.G.: A comparative trial of doxycycline and ampicillin in the treatment of acute sinusitis. Chemotherapy 21 (Suppl. 1): 68-75 (1975).

American Academy of Pediatrics, Committee on Drugs: Requiem for tetracyclines. Pediatrics 55: 142-143 (1975).

American Thoracic Society: Guidelines for work for patients with tuberculosis. American Review of Respiratory Diseases 108: 160-161 (1973).

American Thoracic Society: Treatment of mycobacterial diseases. American Review of Respiratory Diseases 115: 185-187 (1977).

Axelsson, A. and Brorson, J.-E.: Concentrations of antibiotics in sinus secretions: Doxycycline and spiramycin. Annals of Otology, Rhinology and Laryngology 82: 44-48 (1973).

Axelsson, A. and Brorson, J.-E.: Concentrations of antibiotics in sinus secretions: Ampicillin, cephradine and erythromycin estolate. Annals of Otology, Rhinology and Laryngology 83: 323-332 (1974).

Badr-El-Din, M.K.; Aref, G.H.; Kassem, A.S.; Abdel-Moneim, M.A. and Abbassy, A.A.: A beta-adrenergic receptor stimulant, salbutamol, in the treatment of pertussis. Journal of Tropical Medicine and Hygiene 79: 218-219 (1976a).

Badr-El-Din, M.K.; Aref, G.H.; Mazloum, H.; El-Towesy, Y.A.; Kassem, A.S.; Abdel-Moneim, M.A. and Abbassy, A.A.: The beta-adrenergic receptors in pertussis. Journal of Tropical Medicine and Hygiene 79: 213-217 (1966).

Balagtas, R.C.; Nelson, K.E.; Levin, S. and Gotoff, S.P.: Treatment of pertussis with pertussis immune globulin. Journal of Pediatrics 79: 203-208 (1971).

Baraff, L.J.; Wilkins, J. and Wehrle, P.F.: The role of antibiotics, immunizations and adenoviruses in pertussis. Pediatrics 61: 224-230 (1978).

Barrett-Connor, E.: The nonvalue of sputum culture in the diagnosis of pneumococcal pneumonia. American Review of Respiratory Diseases 103: 845-848 (1971).

Bartlett, J.G.; Alexander, J.; Mayhew, J.; Sullivan-Sigler, N. and Gorbach, S.L.: Should fiberoptic bronchoscopy aspirates be cultured? American Review of Respiratory Diseases 114: 73-78 (1976).

Bass, J.W.; Klenk, E.L.; Kotheimer, J.B.; Linnemann, C.C. and Smith, M.H.D.: Antimicrobial treatment of pertussis. Journal of Pediatrics 75: 768-781 (1969).

Bass, J.W.; Podgore, J.K. and Fischer, G.W.: Techniques for recovery of *B. pertussis* on culture. Journal of Pediatrics 87: 670-671 (1975).

Bass, J.W.; Steele, R.W. and Wiebe, R.A.: Acute epiglottitis — a surgical emergency. Journal of the American Medical Association 229: 671-675 (1974).

Bates, J.H. and Stead, W.W.: Effect of chemotherapy on infectiousness of tuberculosis. New England Journal of Medicine 290: 459-460 (1974).

Battaglia, J.D. and Lockhart, C.H.: Management of acute epiglottitis by nasotracheal intubation. American Journal of Diseases of Children 129: 334-336 (1975).

Baxter, J.D.: Acute epiglottitis in children. Laryngoscope 77: 1358-1367 (1967).

Bechamps, G.J.; Lynn, H.B. and Wenzl, J.E.: Empyema in children: Review of Mayo Clinic experience. Mayo Clinic Proceedings 45: 43-50 (1970).

Beem, M.O. and Saxon, E.M.: Respiratory-tract colonization and a distinctive pneumonia syndrome in infants infected with *Chlamydia trachomatis*. N. Engl. J. Med. 296: 306-310 (1977a).

Beem, M.O. and Saxon, E.M.: Uncertainties in the treatment of chlamydial infections in infants. New England Journal of Medicine 296: 1124 (1977b).

Bell, S.M. and Smith, D.D.: Quantitative throat swab culture in the diagnosis of streptococcal pharyngitis in children. Lancet 2: 61-63 (1976).

Benjamin, B. and Dorman, D.: Acute otitis media. Medical Journal of Australia 1: 491-494 (1977).

Berenberg, W. and Kevy, S.: Acute epiglottitis in childhod. A serious emergency readily recognized at the bedside. New England Journal of Medicine 258: 870-874 (1958).

Bland, R.D.: Otitis media in the first six weeks of life: Diagnosis, bacteriology and management. Pediatrics 49: 187-197 (1972).

Bluestone, C.D. and Beery, Q.C.: Concepts on the pathogenesis of middle ear effusions. Annals of Otology, Rhinology and Laryngology 83 (Suppl. 25): 182-186 (1976).

Bluestone, C.D. and Shurin, P.A.: Middle ear disease in children. Pathogenesis, diagnosis and management. Pediatric Clinics of North America 21: 379-400 (1974).

Branefors-Helander, P. and Jeppsson, P.-H.: Acute epiglottitis: A clinical, bacteriological and serological study. Scandinavian Journal of Infectious Diseases 7: 103-111 (1975).

Breese, B.B.; Disney, F.A.; Talpey, W. and Green, J.D.: Beta-hemolytic streptococcal infection: The clinical and epidemiologic importance of the number of organisms found in cultures. American Journal of Diseases of Children 119: 18-26 (1970).

Brewin, A.; Arango, L.; Hadley, W.K. and Murray, J.F.: High-dose penicillin therapy and pneumococcal pneumonia. Journal of the American Medical Association 230: 409-413 (1974).

Brickman, H.F.; Beaudry, P.H. and Marks, M.I.: The timing of tuberculin tests in relation to immunization with live viral vaccines. Pediatrics 55: 392-396 (1975).

British Thoracic and Tuberculosis Association: Short course chemotherapy in pulmonary tuberculosis. Lancet 1: 119-124 (1975) and 2: 1102-1104 (1976).

Brook, I.; Anthony, B. and Finegold, S.M.: Aerobic and anaerobic bacteriology of acute otitis media in children. Paper presented to the 16th Interscience Conference on Antimicrobial Agents and Chemotherapy, Chicago, Illinois, October 28, 1976.

Cameron, G.C.; Pomahac, A.C. and Johnston, M.T.: Comparative efficacy of ampicillin and trimethoprim-sulfamethoxazole in otitis media. Canadian Medical Association Journal 112 (Suppl.): 87S (1975).

Carenfelt, C.; Eneroth, C.-M.; Lundberg, C. and Wretlind, B.: Evaluation of the antibiotic effect of treatment of maxillary sinusitis. Scandinavian Journal of Infectious Diseases 7: 259-264 (1975).

Carr, D.T.: Diagnostic studies of pleural fluid. Surgical Clinics of North America 53: 801-804 (1973).

Cattaneo, S.M. and Kilman, J.W.: Surgical therapy of empyema in children. Archives of Surgery 106: 564-567 (1973).

Caughey, J.E.: Pleuropericardial lesion in Q-fever. British Medical Journal 1: 1447 (1977).

Center for Disease Control, US Public Health Service: Chloramphenicol-resistant *Haemophilus influenzae*. Morbidity and Mortality Weekly Report 25: 267 and 385 (1976).

Ceruti, E.; Conteras, J. and Neira, M.: Staphylococcal pneumonia in childhood. Long-term follow-up including pulmonary function studies. Am. J. Dis. Child. 122: 386-392 (1971).

Chamovitz, R.; Catanzaro, F.J.; Stetson, C.A. and Rammelkamp, C.H.: Prevention of rheumatic fever by treatment of previous streptococcal infections. I. Evaluation of benzathine penicillin G. New England Journal of Medicine 251: 466-471 (1954).

Chandler, J.R.; Langenbrunner, D.J. and Stevens, E.R.: The pathogenesis of orbital complications in acute sinusitis. Laryngoscope 80: 1414-1428 (1970).

Coleman, D.J.: Reliability of ocular and orbital diagnosis with B-scan ultrasound. 2. Orbital diagnosis. American Journal of Ophthalmology 74: 704-718 (1972).

Connor, J.D.: Evidence for an etiologic role of adenoviral infections in pertussis syndrome. New England Journal of Medicine 283: 390-394 (1970).

Davidson, M.; Tempest, B. and Palmer, D.L.: Bacteriologic diagnosis of acute pneumonia. Comparison of sputum, transtracheal aspirates and lung aspirates. Journal of the American Medical Association 235: 158-163 (1976).

Denny, F.W.; Clyde, W.A. and Glezen, W.P.: *Mycoplasma pneumoniae* disease: Clinical Spectrum, pathophysiology, epidemiology and control. Journal of Infectious Diseases 123: 74-92 (1971).

Derrick, C.W. and Dillon, H.C.: Erythromycin therapy for streptococcal pharyngitis. American Journal of Diseases of Children 130: 175-178 (1976).

Deveikis, A.; Schauf, V.; Mizen, M. and Riff, L.: Antimicrobial therapy of experimental group B streptococcal infection in mice. Antimicrobial Agents and Chemotherapy 11: 817-820 (1977).

Dieu, J.-Cl.; Adnis-Lamarre, F.; Bitar, M. and Dabbagh, M.: La rifampicine dans le traitement des formes ganglio-pulmonaires de la tuberculose initiale du nourrisson et de l'enfant. Revue de la Tuberculose et de Pneumonologie 34: 320-331 (1970).

Doster, B.; Nurray, F.J. and Newman, R.: Ethambutol in the initial treatment of pulmonary tuberculosis. American Review of Respiratory Diseases 107: 177-190 (1973).

Dunbar, J.S.: Epiglottitis and croup. J. Can. Assoc. Radiol. 12: 86-95 (1961).

Eavey, R.D.; Stool, S.E.; Peckham, G.J. and Mitchell, L.R.: How to examine the ear of the neonate. Clinical Pediatrics 15: 338-341 (1976).

Editorial: BCG and the tuberculin test. Lancet 1: 192-193 (1969).

Editorial: Ear drops. Lancet 1: 896 (1976).

Evans, F.O. Jr.; Sydnor, J.B.; Moore, W.E.C.; Moore, G.R.; Manwaring, J.L.; Brill, A.H.; Jackson, R.T.; Hanna, S.; Skarr, J.S.; Holdeman, L.V.; Fitz-Hugh, G.S.; Sande, M.A. and Gwaltney, J.M. Jr.: Sinusitis of the maxillary antrum. New England Journal of Medicine 293: 735-739 (1975).

Feigin, R.D.; Shackelford, P.G.; Campbell, J.; Lyles, T.O.; Schechter, M. and Lins, R.D.: Assessment of the role of Staphylococcus epidermidis as a cause of otitis media. Pediatrics 52: 569-576 (1973).

Ferebee, S.H.: Controlled chemoprophylaxis trials in tuberculosis: A general review. Advances in Tuberculosis Research (Bibliotheca Tuberculosea No. 26) 17: 28-106 (1970).

Fernald, G.W.; Collier, A.M. and Clyde, W.A.: Respiratory infections due to Mycoplasma pneumoniae in infants and children. Pediatrics 55: 327-335 (1975).

Fine, M.L.; Smith, L.R. and Sheedy, P.F.: Frequency of pleural effusions in mycoplasma and viral pneumonias. New England Journal of Medicine 283: 790-793 (1970).

Foy, H.M.; Cooney, M.K.; McMahan, R. and Grayston, J.T.: Viral and mycoplasmal pneumonia in a Prepaid Medical Care Group during an eight-year period. American Journal of Epidemiology 97: 93-102 (1973).

Friedberg, J.: Maxillary sinus disease and the pediatric patient. Otolaryngiologic Clinics of North America 9: 163-173 (1976).

Gellady, A.M.; Shulman, S.T. and Ayoub, E.M.: Orbital cellulitis in children. Pediatric Research 11: 500 (Abstract No. 769) (1977).

Geraci, R.P.: Acute epiglottitis — management with prolonged nasotracheal intubation. Pediatrics 41: 143-145 (1968).

Gerbeaux, J.; Hanoteau, J. and Couvreur, J.: New drugs in primary tuberculosis in children. Pediatrics Digest 17: 22-29 (June, 1975).

Girling, D.J.: Adverse reactions to rifampicin in antituberculosis regimens. Journal of Antimicrobial Chemotherapy 3: 115-132 (1977).

Glezen, W.P. and Denny, F.W.: Epidemiology of acute lower respiratory diesase in children. New England Journal of Medicine 288: 498-505 (1973).

Grix, A. and Giammona, S.T.: Pneumonitis with pleural effusion in children due to Mycoplasma pneumoniae. American Review of Respiratory Diseases 109: 665-671 (1974).

Grossman, E.R.; Walchek, A. and Freedman, H.: Tetracyclines and permanent teeth: The relation between dose and tooth color. Pediatrics 47: 567-570 (1971).

Gunnels, J.J.; Bates, J.H. and Swindoll, H.: Infectivity of sputum positive tuberculosis patients on chemotherapy. American Review of Respiratory Diseases 109: 323-330 (1974).

Harrison, H.R.; English, M.G.; Lee, C.K. and Alexander, E.R.: Chlamydia trachomatis infant pneumonitis: Comparison with matched controls and other infant pneumonitis. New England Journal of Medicine 298: 702-708 (1978).

Hawkins, D.B. and Clark, R.W.: Orbital involvement in acute sinusitis. Lessons from 24 childhood patients. Clinical Pediatrics 16: 464-471 (1977).

Haynes, R.E. and Cramblett, H.G.: Acute ethmoiditis: Its relationship to orbital cellulitis. American Journal of Diseases of Children 114: 261-267 (1967).

Hemming, V.G.; McCloskey, D.W. and Hill, H.R.: Pneumonia in the neonate associated with group B streptococcal septicemia. American Journal of Diseases of Children 130: 1231-1233 (1976).

Holm, V.A. and Kunze, L.H.: Effect of chronic otitis media on language and speech development. Pediatrics 43: 833-839 (1969).

Honig, P.J.; Pasquariello, P.S. and Stool, S.E.: *H. influenzae* pneumonia in infants and children. Journal of Pediatrics 83: 215-219 (1973).

Howard, J.E.; Nelson, J.D.; Clahsen, J. and Jackson, L.H.: Otitis media of infancy and early childhood: A double-blind study of four treatment regimens. American Journal of Diseases of Children 130: 965-970 (1976).

Howie, V.M.; Ploussard, H.J. and Lester, R.L.: Otitis media: A clinical and bacteriological correlation. Pediatrics 45: 29-35 (1970).

Howie, V.M.; Ploussard, J.H. and Sloyer, J.: Comparison of ampicillin and amoxicillin in the treatment of otitis media in children. Journal of Infectious Diseases 129 (Suppl.): S181-S184 (1974).

Howie, V.M.; Ploussard, J.H. and Sloyer, J.L.: Immunization against recurrent otitis media. Annals of Otology, Rhinology and Laryngology 85 (Suppl. 25): 254-258 (1976).

Hsu, K.H.K.: Isoniazid in the prevention and treatment of tuberculosis: A 20-year study of the effectiveness in children. Journal of the American Medical Association 229: 528-533 (1974).

Irwin, R.S.; Seith, W.F.; Woelk, W.K. and Enegren, B.J.: Cell wall-deficient bacterial variant cultural surveillance: A useful laboratory aid. American Journal of Medicine 59: 129-133 (1975).

Johnson, G.K.; Sullivan, J.L. and Bishop, L.A.: Acute epiglottitis: Review of 55 cases and suggested protocol. Archives of Otolaryngology 100: 333-337 (1974).

Johnston, R.F. and Wildrick, K.H.: "State of the Art" review. The impact of chemotherapy on the care of patients with tuberculosis. American Review of Respiratory Diseases 109: 646-664 (1974).

Joncas, J.H.; Robitaille, R. and Gauthier, T.: Interpretation of the PPD skin test in BCG-vaccinated children. Canadian Medical Association Journal 113: 127-128 (1975).

Kamme, C.; Lundgren, K. and Mardh, P.-A.: The aetiology of acute otitis media in children. Scandinavian Journal of Infectious Diseases 3: 217-223 (1971).

Kaplan, E.L.; Top, F.H.; Dudding, B.A. and Wannamaker, L.W.: Diagnosis of streptococcal pharyngitis: Differentiation of active infection from the carrier state in the symptomatic child. Journal of Infectious Diseases 123: 490-501 (1971).

Kendig, E.L.: Tuberculosis; in Kendig (Ed) Disorders of the Respiratory Tract in Children, Chapter 46, pp.642-695 (Saunders, Philadelphia 1972).

Khan, W.N.; Rodriguez, W.; Controni, G. and Ross, S.: Incidence of ampicillin-resistant Haemophilus species and synergistic effect of an erythromycin-sulfamethoxazole combination against them. Paper presented to the 16th Interscience Conference on Antimicrobial Agents and Chemotherapy, Chicago, Illinois, Oct. 27, 1976.

Klein, J.O. and Teele, D.W.: Isolation of viruses and mycoplasmas from middle ear effusions: A Review. Annals of Otology, Rhinology and Laryngology 85 (Suppl. 25): 140-144 (1976).

Klimek, J.J.; Nightingale, C.; Lehmann, W.B. and Quintiliani, R.: Comparison of concentrations of amoxicillin and ampicillin in serum and middle ear fluid of children with chronic otitis media. Journal of Infectious Diseases 135: 999-1002 (1977).

Kogutt, M.S. and Swischuk, L.E.: Diagnosis of sinusitis in infants and children. Pediatrics 52: 121-124 (1973).

Kutnick, S.L. and Kerth, J.D.: Acute sinusitis and otitis: Their complications and surgical treatment. Otolaryngological Clinics of North America 9: 689-701 (1976).

Landau, L.I.: Treatment of bronchitis in childhood. Drugs 16: (1978).

Lincoln, E.M. and Sewell, E.M.: Tuberculosis; in Krugman et al. (Eds.) Infectious Diseases of Children 6th Ed, Chapter 31, pp.389-450 (Mosby, St. Louis 1977).

Linnemann, C.C.; Partin, J.C.; Perlstein, P.H. and Englender, G.S.: Pertussis: Persistent problems. Journal of Pediatrics 85: 589-591 (1974).

Linnemann, C.C.; Ramundo, N.; Perlstein, P.H.; Minton, S.D.; Englender, G.S.; McCormick, J.B. and Hayes, P.S.: Use of pertussis vaccine in an epidemic involving hospital staff. Lancet 2: 540-543 (1975).

McGowan, J.E.; Terry, P.M. and Nahmias, A.J.: Susceptibility of *Haemophilus influenzae* isolates from blood and cerebrospinal fluid to ampicillin, chloramphenicol and trimethoprim-sulfamethoxazole. Antimicrobial Agents and Chemotherapy 9: 137-139 (1976).

McLinn, S.E.; Daly, J.F. and Jones, J.E.: Cephalexin monohydrate suspension: Treatment of otitis media. Journal of the American Medical Association 234: 171-173 (1975).

Margolis, C.Z.; Colletti, R.B. and Grundy, G.: *Hemophilus influenzae* type B: The etiologic agent in epiglottitis. Journal of Pediatrics 87: 322-323 (1975).

Markowitz, M. and Gordis, L.: Rheumatic fever — primary prevention; in Rheumatic Fever, Vol. 11, Major Problems in Clinical Pediatrics, 2nd Ed. (Saunders, Philadelphia 1972).

Marks, M.I.: In vitro activity of clindamycin and other antimicrobials against Gram-positive bacteria and *Hemophilus influenzae*. Canadian Medical Association Journal 112: 170-173 (1975).

Mason, W.H.; Siegel, S.E. and Tucker, B.L.: Diagnostic open lung biopsy in children. Pediatric Research 11: 503 (Abstract No. 787) [1977].

Miller, C.L.; Pollock, T.M. and Jones, A.D.E.: Whooping-cough vaccination: An assessment. Lancet 2: 510-513 (1974).

Mimica, I.; Donoso, E.; Howard, J.E. and Ledermann, G.W.: Lung puncture in etiological diagnosis of pneumonia. American Journal of Diseases of Children 122: 278-282 (1971).

Molteni, R.A.: Epiglottitis: Incidence of extraepiglottic infection. Report of 72 cases and review of the literature. Pediatrics 58: 526-531 (1971).

Murray, P.R. and Washington, J.J.II.: Microscopic and bacteriologic analysis of expectorated sputum. Mayo Clinic Proceedings 50: 339-344 (1975).

Nelson, K.E.; Gavitt, F.; Batt, M.D.; Kallick, C.A.; Reddi, K.T. and Levin, S.: The role of adenoviruses in the pertussis syndrome. Journal of Pediatrics 86: 335 (1975).

Neu, H.C.: Antimicrobial activity and human pharmacology of amoxicillin. Journal of Infectious Diseases 129 (Suppl.): S123-S131 (1974).

Newman, R.; Doster, B.E.; Murray, F.J. and Woolpert, S.F.: Rifampin in initial treatment of pulmonary tuberculosis. American Review of Respiratory Diseases 109: 216-232 (1974).

Noah, N.D.: Attack rates of notified whooping cough in immunised and unimmunised children. British Medical Journal 1: 128-129 (1976).

Paradise, J.L.: On tympanostomy tubes: Rationale, results, reservations and recommendations. Pediatrics 60: 86-90 (1977).

Parrott, R.H.; Vargosko, A.J.; Kim, H.W.; Bell, J.A. and Chanock, R.M.: Respiratory diseases of viral etiology. 3. Myxoviruses: parainfluenza. American Journal of Public Health 52: 907 (1962).

Perrin, J.M.: Management of recurrent otitis media. New England Journal of Medicine 291: 1364 (1974).

Perrin, J.M.; Charney, E.; MacWhinney, J.B.; McInerny, T.K.; Miller, R.L. and Nazarian, L.F.: Sulfisox-azole as chemoprophylaxis for recurrent otitis media. New England Journal of Medicine 291: 664-667 (1974).

Pilheu, J.A.: Short-duration treatment of pulmonary tuberculosis. Chest 71: 583-586 (1977).

Potter, A.R. and Fischer, G.W.: *Haemophilus influenzae*, the predominant cause of bacterial pneumonia in Hawaii. Pediatric Research 11: 504 (Abstr. 795) [1977].

Preston, N.W.: Protection by pertussis vaccine — little cause for concern. Lancet 1: 1065-1067 (1976).

Preston, N.W. and Stanbridge, T.N.: Whooping-cough vaccination. Lancet 1: 1089 (1975).

Quick, C.A.: Comparison of penicillin and trimethoprim-sulfamethoxazole in the treatment of ear, nose and throat infections. Canadian Medical Association Journal 112 (Suppl): 83S (1975).

Quick, C.A. and Payne, E.: Complicated acute sinusitis. Laryngoscope 82: 1248-1263 (1972).

Quinn, R.W.; Denny, F.W. and Riley, H.D.: Natural occurrence of hemolytic streptococci in normal school children. American Journal of Public Health 47: 995-1008 (1957).

Quinn, R.W. and Federspiel, C.F.: The incidence of rheumatic fever in metropolitan Nashville, 1963-69. American Journal of Epidemiology 99: 273-280 (1974).

Rapkin, R.H.: Tracheostomy in epiglottitis, Pediatrics 52: 426-429 (1973).

Ravitch, M.M. and Fein, R.: The changing picture of pneumonia and empyema in infants and children. Journal of the American Medical Association 175: 1039-1044 (1961).

Riley, H.D. and Bracken, E.C.: Empyema due to *H. influenzae* in infants and children. American Journal of Diseases of Children 110: 24-28 (1965).

Robins, J. and Fitz-Hugh, G.: Epiglottitis in the adult. Laryngoscope 81: 700-706 (1971).

Ross, P.W.: Beta-hemolytic streptococci in saliva. Journal of Hygiene 69: 347-353 (1971).

Rowe, D.S.: Acute suppurative otitis media. Pediatrics 56: 285-294 (1975).

Schauf, V.; Deveikis, A.; Riff, L. and Serota, A.: Antibiotic-killing kinetics of group B streptococci. Journal of Pediatrics 89: 194-198 (1976).

Schwartz, R.; Rodriguez, W.J.; Khan, W.N. and Ross, S.: Acute purulent otitis media in children older than 5 years. Incidence of *Haemophilus* as a causative organism. Journal of the American Medical Association 238: 1032-1033 (1977).

Schwartz, R.; Rodriguez, W.; Khan, W. and Ross, S.: The increasing incidence of ampicillin-resistant *Haemophilus influenzae*. Journal of the American Medical Association 239: 320-323 (1978).

Sewell, E.M.; O'Hare, D. and Kendig, E.L.: The tuberculin test. Pediatrics 54: 650-653 (1974).

Shurin, P.A.; Pelton, S.I. and Finkelstein, J.: Tympanometry in the diagnosis of middle-ear effusion. New England Journal of Medicine 296: 412-417 (1977).

Shurin, P.A.; Pelton, S.I. and Klein, J.O.: Otitis media in the newborn infant. Annals of Otology, Rhinology and Laryngology 85 (Suppl. 25): 216-222 (1976).

Shurin, P.A.; Pelton, S.I.; Scheifele, D. and Klein, J.O.: Otitis media caused by non-typable, ampicillin-resistant strains of *Haemophilus influenzae*. Journal of Pediatrics 88: 646-649 (1976).

Shuttleworth, D.B. and Charney, E.: Leukocyte count in childhood pneumonia. American Journal of Diseases of Children 122: 393-396 (1971).

Simon, K.: Rifampicin behandlung der tuberkulose im kindesalter (therapy of tuberculosis with rifampicin in childhood). Medizinische Klinik 70: 1095-1097 (1975).

Sloyer, J.L.; Cate, C.C.; Howie, V.M.; Ploussard, J.H. and Johnston, R.B.: Immune response to acute otitis media in children. 2. Serum and middle ear fluid antibody in otitis media due to *H. influenzae*. Journal of Infectious Diseases 132: 685-688 (1975).

Sloyer, J.L.; Howie, I.M.; Ploussard, J.H.; Ammann, A.J.; Austrian, R. and Johnston, R.B.: The immune response to acute otitis media in childhood. 1. Serotypes isolated and serum and middle ear fluid antibody in pneumococcal otitis media. Infection and Immunity 9: 1028-1032 (1974).

Smilack, J.D.; Burgin, W.W.; Moore, W.L. and Sanford, J.P.: *Mycoplasma pneumoniae* pneumonia and clindamycin therapy: Failure to demonstrate efficacy. Journal of the American Medical Association 228: 729-731 (1974).

Smith, A.L.: Antibiotics and invasive *Haemophilus influenzae*. New England Journal of Medicine 294: 1329-1331 (1976).

Stechenberg, B.W.; Anderson, D.; Chang, M.J.; Dunkle, L.; Wong, M.; van Reken, D.; Pickering, L.K. and Feigin, R.D.: Cephalexin compared to ampicillin treatment of otitis media. Pediatrics 58: 532-536 (1976).

Strome, M. and Jaffe, B.: Epiglottitis — individualized management with steroids. Laryngoscope 84: 921-928 (1974).

Stuart-Harris, C.H. (chairman, Joint Committee of Vaccination and Immunization of the Central Health Services Council and the Scottish Health Service Planning Council): Statement on whooping cough vaccine. British Medical Journal 3: 687-688 (1975).

Syriopoulou, V.; Scheifele, D.; Howie, V.; Ploussard, J.; Sloyer, J. and Smith, A.L.: Incidence of ampicillin-resistant *Hemophilus influenzae* in otitis media. Journal of Pediatrics 89: 839-841 (1976).

Taussig, L.M.; Belmonte, M.M. and Beaudry, P.H.: *Staphylococcus aureus* empyema in cystic fibrosis. Journal of Pediatrics 84: 724-727 (1974).

Tetzlaff, T.R.; Ashworth, C. and Nelson, J.D.: Otitis media in children less than 12 weeks of age. Pediatrics 59: 827-832 (1977).

van de Water, J.M.: The treatment of pleural effusion complicating pneumonia. Chest 57: 259-262 (1970).

van Overbeek, J.J.M.: Gonorrheal infections in the oropharynx. Archives of Otolaryngology 102: 94-96 (1976).

Vollman, J.H.; Smith, W.L.; Ballard, E.T. and Light, I.J.: Early onset group B streptococcal disease: Clinical, roentgenographic and pathologic features. Journal of Pediatrics 89: 199-203 (1976).

Watters, E.C.; Wallar, P.H.; Hiles, D.A. and Michaels, R.H.: Acute orbital cellulitis. Archives of Ophthalmology 94: 785-788 (1976).

Weber, M.J.; Desjardins, R.; Perreault, G.; Rivard, G. and Turmel, Y.: Acute epiglottitis in children — treatment with nasotracheal intubation: Report of 14 consecutive cases. Pediatrics 57: 153-155 (1976).

Wilkins, J. and Bass, J.W.: Pertussis; in Top and Wehrle (Eds.) Communicable and Infectious Diseases 8th Ed, pp.491-501 (Mosby, St. Louis 1976).

Wise, M.R.; Beaudry, P.H. and Bates, D.V.: Long-term follow-up of staphylococcal pneumonia. Pediatrics 38: 398-401 (1977).

Wise, P.J. and Neu, H.C.: Experience with amoxicillin: An overall summary of clinical trials in the United States. Journal of Infectious Diseases 129 (Suppl): S266-S271 (1974).

Wolff, L.J.; Bartlett, M.S.; Baehner, R.L.; Grosfeld, J.L. and Smith, J.W.: The causes of interstitial pneumonitis in immunocompromised children: An aggressive systematic approach to diagnosis. Pediatrics 60: 41-45 (1977).

Wright, J.E.; Lloyd, G.A.S. and Ambrose, J.: Computerized axial tomography in the detection of orbital space occupying lesions. American Journal of Ophthalmology 80: 78-84 (1975).

Zanen, H.C.; Ganor, S. and van Toorn, M.J.: Continuous study of hemolytic streptococci in the throats of normal children, adults and aged men. American Journal of Hygiene 69: 265-273 (1959).

Zimmerman, R.A.; Horn, K.A.; Meyer, W.T. and Klesius, P.H.: Applying an old concept to a new method of streptococcal surveillance. Pediatrics 53: 275-279 (1974).

Zollar, L.M.; Krause, H.E. and Mufson, M.A.: Microbiologic studies on young infants with lower respiratory tract diseases. American Journal of Diseases of Children 126: 56-60 (1973).

Chapter III

Infections of the Central Nervous System

G.A. Ahronheim

All varieties of organism are capable of causing central nervous system (CNS) infections (Bell and McCormick, 1975). This chapter will be limited to some of the more common and important bacterial infections of the CNS in infants and children, with emphasis on current concepts in therapy.

1. Pyogenic Meningitis

Acute bacterial meningitis takes several distinct forms in children — neonatal meningitis, purulent meningitis of childhood, and tuberculous meningitis — each with its characteristic clinical manifestations, therapeutic requirements and prognosis.

1.1 Neonatal Meningitis

Meningitis occurring in the first few weeks of life is usually part of a generalised sepsis syndrome, with non-specific presenting signs. Despite many advances in supportive and antibiotic therapy, the morbidity and mortality of neonatal meningitis remain high (Bell and McCormick, 1975; Bortolussi et al., 1978). Other aspects of neonatal sepsis are discussed in detail in chapter VIII.

1.1.1 Pathogenic Organisms

The most common pathogens are the enteric Gram-negative bacilli, particularly *Escherichia coli*. Since 1970, Lancefield group B streptococci *(Streptococcus agalactiae)* have become increasingly recognised as the next most frequent cause of sepsis neonatorum (Barton et al., 1973), and in some studies have apparently surpassed *E. coli* (Baker et al., 1973). Less frequently encountered are *Staphylococcus aureus, Pseudomonas aeruginosa*, the pneumococcus and *Listeria monocytogenes*.

1.1.2 Treatment

Pending results of cultures, antibiotic therapy for neonatal sepsis and meningitis is usually initiated with a combination of a β-lactam antibiotic (the penicillins) and an aminoglycoside (e.g. kanamycin, gentamicin, etc). Many enteric Gram-negative bacilli are often resistant to the concentrations of β-lactam drugs ordinarily achieved in the cerebrospinal fluid (CSF), but combination with an aminoglycoside is frequently synergistic. The initial choice of drugs should be made according to local experience of susceptibility patterns and common organisms, and then revised as guided by testing of the patient's isolate. Ampicillin is the recommended β-lactam drug for coliform and Listeria infections. Crystalline penicillin G is the drug of choice for pneumococcal and streptococcal meningitis; however, high doses may be required for group B streptococci (McCracken, 1976), and ampicillin may be preferable for enterococci. Carbenicillin should be reserved for infections due to Pseudomonas and ampicillin-resistant strains of indole-positive Proteus (Hewitt and Winters, 1973), and used only in combination with an appropriate aminoglycoside to prevent the emergence of carbenicillin resistance (Eickhoff and Marks, 1970; Gaman et al., 1976).

Kanamycin and gentamicin have proved very useful against most coliforms, but the emergence of resistant organisms — generally related to the intensity of use of the drug in question (Howard and McCracken, 1975a) — emphasises the necessity of monitoring trends in local susceptibility patterns. Numerous variables including gestational age, body weight, renal function, etc. affect antibiotic pharmacokinetics dramatically in the newborn period (McCracken, 1974; McCracken and Eichenwald, 1974; McCracken and Nelson, 1977; McCracken and Threlkeld, 1976). Recommended dosages in this age group are given in table I.

Route of Administration
We prefer the intravenous (IV) route, especially for β-lactam drugs because:
1) higher peak serum concentrations may be achieved;
2) infants have relatively little muscle mass to absorb intramuscular injections; and
3) absorption of intramuscular drugs may be less reliable in the critically ill patient with unstable peripheral circulation and perfusion.

Because of relatively poor penetration of the so-called blood-brain barrier, the efficacy of parenteral aminoglycosides in infections of the CNS remains problematical (Chang et al., 1975); hence the need for frequent monitoring of the CSF to gauge progress. Although direct instillation of aminoglycosides into the CSF has theoretical

Table I. Dosages of antibacterial agents in central nervous system infections

Drug	Dose	Route
Amikacin	*Neonates:* 15mg/kg/day divided q12h (q8h when weight > 2kg and age > 7d)	IM, IV
Ampicillin	*First week of life:* 50 to 100mg/kg/day divided q12h	IM, IV
	Age 1 week to 1 month: 150 to 200mg/kg/day divided q6 to 8h	IM, IV
	Above 1 month of age: 400mg/kg/day divided q4h	IV
Carbenicillin	*Infants less than 2kg:* 225mg/kg/day divided q8h, up to age 7 days	IV
	Infants greater than 2kg: 300mg/kg/day divided q6h, up to age 4 days	
	Thereafter: 400mg/kg/day divided q4 to q6h	
Chloramphenicol	*Newborn:* 25mg/kg/day once daily during first 2 weeks of life, then 50mg/kg/day divided q12h	IV
	Above 1 month of age: 100mg/kg/day divided q6h	IV
Cloxacillin	100 to 200mg/kg/day divided q6 to 8h	IV
Gentamicin	*Infants less than 2kg:* 5mg/kg/day divided q12 to 24h during 1st week of life, 7.5mg/kg/day divided q12h thereafter	IM, IV
	Infants greater than 2kg: 7.5mg/kg/day divided q12h during 1st week of life, q8h thereafter	IM, IV
	Intraventricular: 1 to 5mg/dose daily until no organisms seen in ventricular fluid	
Isoniazid (INH)	15 to 20mg/kg/day divided q12h	PO
	10mg/kg/day divided q12h	IM
Kanamycin	*Infants less than 2kg:* 15mg/kg/day divided q12h during 1st week of life, 20mg/kg/day divided q12h thereafter	IM, IV
	Infants greater than 2kg: 20mg/kg/day divided q12h 1st week of life, 30mg/kg/day divided q8h thereafter	IM, IV
Methicillin	250 to 300mg/kg/day divided q6h	IV
Nafcillin	150 to 200mg/kg/day divided q6h	IV
Penicillin G	*Neonates:* 50,000 to 100,000u/kg/day divided q12h during the first 4 days of life, then q6 to q8h	IM, IV
	100,000 to 250,000u/kg/day, divided as above, for group B streptococcal sepsis and meningitis	IM, IV
	Older infants and children: 100,000 to 500,000u/kg/day divided q2 to 6h	IV
Tobramycin	*Neonates:* 4 to 6mg/kg/day divided q12h during 1st week of life, q8h thereafter	IM, IV

advantages (Kaiser and McGee, 1975), this remains unproven as a significantly useful manoeuvre in neonates. A recent prospective controlled trial (McCracken and Mize, 1976) found no significant improvement in the overall outcome of enteric Gram-negative infantile meningitis when lumbar intrathecal gentamicin was added to a parenteral ampicillin + gentamicin regimen; this may be due to the frequent co-existence of ventriculitis (Gilles et al., 1977; Yeung, 1976), poor circulation into the ventricles of drug injected into the lumbar subarachnoid space, or perhaps an inadequate (1 mg) intrathecal dose. On the other hand, administration directly into the ventricles, using a subgaleal-ventricular cannula with a subcutaneous reservoir (Salmon, 1972), would take advantage of the physiological circulation of CSF and may prove to be a major advance. In an individual case, if progress is poor and CSF cultures remain positive, the ventricular fluid should be examined and 1 to 5mg gentamicin can be instilled directly at the time of ventricular puncture (McCracken and Nelson, 1977). Although aminoglycosides have generally been well tolerated when injected directly into the CSF, irritation can occur (Hollifield et al., 1976), and preservative-free preparations for intra-CNS administration should be used if available.

Staphylococcal Neonatal Meningitis

This generally requires the use of semisynthetic antistaphylococcal penicillins such as cloxacillin or nafcillin. Although nafcillin, for example, may reach bactericidal levels against staphylococci in the CSF (Kane et al., 1977), these drugs may not always achieve adequate concentrations in the CNS. Thus as with Gram-negative meningitis, therapy should be monitored by demonstrating prompt sterilisation of, and adequate levels or antibacterial activity in, the CSF. Cephalosporins have even more variable and unreliable penetration into the CSF and cannot be recommended without scrupulous monitoring (Fisher et al., 1975). Vancomycin is a potent bactericidal agent against staphylococci, and has been reported to cure staphylococcal meningitis in a dose of 40 to 50mg/kg/24 hours (Hawley and Gump, 1973).

If the chosen therapy does not produce prompt sterilisation of the CSF, we recommend direct instillation into the CSF of gentamicin (to which at least 95% of staphylococci are sensitive) following each daily monitoring tap.

Other Drugs

The emergence of gentamicin resistant strains of *Pseudomonas aeruginosa* (Gaman et al., 1976) and coliforms is another major problem which generally requires the use of newer aminoglycosides such as amikacin, tobramycin or sisomicin. Experience with these drugs in newborns is limited, but where clinical response and susceptibility testing suggest that they may succeed where kanamycin and gentamicin have not, their use may be necessary (Howard and McCracken, 1975b; Kannan et al., 1973; Kaplan et al., 1973; Marks, 1975; Marks et al., 1978).

Chloramphenicol, which achieves relatively good CNS concentrations, may occasionally be useful against sensitive organisms in selected cases. Because of its potential for dose-related toxicity and the 'grey baby syndrome' in the neonate, it is given in reduced doses: 25mg/kg/day in the first two weeks of life. The toxic concentration of chloramphenicol in the serum of neonates is estimated to be above 50µg/ml (of free base); however, various assays yield conflicting results and while serum concentrations should be monitored in neonates, the results do have to be interpreted with caution (McCracken and Nelson, 1977). Intramuscular chloramphenicol is not well absorbed in the active form due to inadequate muscle esterase activity (DuPont et al., 1970) and the drug should therefore be administered IV in serious infections; despite its relatively good absorption orally, inadequate data exist to recommend this route for meningitis.

Duration of Therapy

Antibiotic therapy for neonatal meningitis is usually continued for at least two weeks after the first negative CSF culture, and in most cases for more than three weeks total in this institution.

The optimum duration of intrathecal or intraventricular therapy has not been established, but we recommend that it be continued until a negative culture has been obtained (sterile after 48 hours of incubation) and the clinical status of the baby and the CSF has improved.

1.2 Purulent Meningitis of Childhood

This entity is among the most serious common infections in infants and children.

1.2.1 Pathogenic Organisms

Haemophilus influenzae type b is especially common in the age range of one month to 5 years. The other major pathogens are the pneumococcus *(Streptococcus pneumoniae,* formerly called *Diplococcus pneumoniae)* and the meningococcus *(Neisseria meningitidis)* which are common at all ages and predominate in older children (Goldacre, 1976; Swartz and Dodge, 1965; Yow et al., 1973).

1.2.2 Treatment

For more than a decade, ampicillin has provided effective initial antibiotic therapy for bacterial meningitis in this age group (Mathies, 1972; Yow et al., 1973). However, the appearance of ampicillin resistant strains of *H. influenzae* type b (American Academy of Pediatrics, 1976; Fallon, 1976) has seriously complicated the approach to this disease (Katz, 1975; Smith, 1976), as has the recognition of strains of pneumococci relatively resistant to penicillin (Ahronheim and Marks, 1977; Hansman,

1974; Naraqi et al., 1974). These findings re-emphasise the need for careful laboratory identification and study of bacterial isolates. Testing isolates of *H. influenzae* type b for the production of β-lactamase is a useful rapid means of recognising ampicillin resistant strains, and in our laboratory correlates well with quantitative sensitivity testing (Catlin, 1975; Escamilla, 1976; Jorgensen and Lee, 1975; Marks and Weinmaster, 1975; Thornsberry and Kirven, 1974a,b).

Initial Therapy

High dose IV ampicillin (400mg/kg/day in 4 to 6 divided doses) is recommended for meningitis in children up to six years of age, pending identification of the organism. In areas where ampicillin resistant strains of *H. influenzae* type b have been recognised, or where appropriate study of *H. influenzae* type b isolates cannot be performed, chloramphenicol (100mg/kg/day in 4 divided doses IV) should be added to the initial ampicillin therapy (American Academy of Pediatrics, 1976). *In vitro* data indicate that the combination of chloramphenicol with either ampicillin or penicillin is not less effective than either drug alone against *H. influenzae* type b — i.e. antagonism is not observed (Ahronheim, 1975; Feldman, 1978). However, studies in experimental pneumococcal meningitis suggest that doses of the β-lactam drug should precede, rather than follow, doses of chloramphenicol (Wallace et al., 1967).

If an ampicillin sensitive *H. influenzae* type b is isolated, chloramphenicol should be discontinued; if the strain is ampicillin resistant (minimum inhibitory concentration > 2μg/ml) and/or β-lactamase positive, ampicillin should be stopped and chloramphenicol continued alone.

If a pneumococcus or meningococcus is isolated, therapy should be changed to penicillin G alone in a dose of 100,000 to 200,000 units/kg/day in 4 to 6 divided doses IV; this is the initial therapy of choice in older children, in whom these organisms predominate and *H. influenzae* type b is relatively uncommon.

Duration of Therapy

Antibiotics are continued intravenously and in full doses (Smith et al., 1973) until the child has been clinically satisfactory and afebrile for at least five days, with a normal peripheral white cell count and CSF findings returning to normal; the minimum duration of treatment recommended is seven days.

1.3 Tuberculous Meningitis

Because of its insidious onset, tuberculous meningitis is frequently unrecognised until florid CNS signs appear, by which time its prognosis has begun to worsen significantly (Idriss et al., 1976; Smith, 1975; Sumaya et al., 1975). A high index of suspicion, careful clinical history, microbiological study, tuberculin skin tests and chest radiography are vital to early diagnosis.

1.3.1 Treatment

Antimicrobial therapy, which should not be deferred pending culture results in a suspected case of tuberculous meningitis, has included three major agents:

1) Isoniazid (INH), 20mg/kg/day orally in 2 or 3 divided doses (or if parenteral treatment is required, 10mg/kg/day IM in two divided doses) for 4 to 6 weeks, followed by 10mg/kg/day orally for 18 to 24 months.

2) Para-aminosalicylic acid (PAS), 200 to 300mg/kg/day in 4 divided doses by mouth or gastric tube for 18 to 24 months.

3) Streptomycin, 30 to 40mg/kg/day IM in one or two divided doses for up to 8 weeks after satisfactory clinical and laboratory improvement have occurred.

In recent years, rifampicin has been found to be a highly effective antituberculous drug and may eventually supplant streptomycin and PAS for the treatment of tuberculous meningitis (Sifontes, 1975). A recent clinical trial in Thailand (Visudhiphan and Chiemchanya, 1975) found rifampicin (15mg/kg/day orally before breakfast) plus isoniazid to yield better results in the treatment of tuberculous meningitis than the traditional isoniazid + PAS + streptomycin regimen.

1.3.2 Treatment of Resistant Strains

The clinician must be alert to the possibility of drug resistant strains of *Mycobacterium tuberculosis;* if the probable contact of the case is known and if that person's organism has already been studied, presumptive data regarding drug susceptibility may be available long before the patient's organism appears in culture. Although experience in children is limited and toxicity difficult to monitor, ethambutol (15mg/kg/day) may be added to initial therapy when a resistant organism is suspected (Steiner and Portugaleza, 1973).

2. Brain Abscess

Brain abscesses in children are most commonly related to cyanotic congenital heart disease (Fischbein et al., 1974), as well as to bacteraemia of any cause or to suppurative infection of the ear and paranasal sinuses.

2.1 Pathogenic Organisms

The wide variety of organisms found reflects the original source of infection. α-Haemolytic *Streptococcus viridans* and other aerobic respiratory tract flora have been commonly described in paediatric cardiac patients (Fischbein et al., 1974); anaerobic bacteria are especially common in infections of the paranasal sinuses (Frederick and Braude, 1974), and the importance of these organisms, hitherto probably greatly under reported, has become increasingly recognised and emphasised as anaerobic culture methods have improved (Heineman and Braude, 1963; Yoshikawa and Goodman, 1974).

2.2 Treatment

Antibiotic therapy of brain abscess seems to serve principally by arresting the progress of the cerebritic process surrounding the lesion, contributing to the walling-off of the abscess by assisting host defence mechanisms. Primary sterilisation by antibiotics alone is uncommon, due to either inadequate concentrations of drug in the abscess cavity, or to decreased drug activity in pus despite seemingly adequate levels (Black et al., 1973). A recent report of sterilisation of a brain abscess with co-trimoxazole, with demonstration of bactericidal concentrations in the abscess fluid, is of considerable interest and deserves further attention (Greene et al., 1975).

As the majority of abscesses are caused by penicillin sensitive organisms (i.e. aerobic and anaerobic streptococci, and most other anaerobes except *Bacteroides fragilis)*, the use of high dose penicillin G therapy is justified in patients with cyanotic congenital heart disease, otitic or sinus disease, and those with no obvious predisposing cause. Chloramphenicol is also widely used because of its relatively good penetration into the CNS and because of its good spectrum against most anaerobes, including *B. fragilis*. A combination of penicillin and chloramphenicol is therefore frequently recommended for initial therapy.

Metronidazole is active against many anaerobes, including *B. fragilis*, and may penetrate into the CSF (Ingham et al., 1977); this drug merits further study with controlled clinical trials in brain abscess.

2.3 Adjunctive Therapy

Acute management of brain abscess should also include control of intracranial hypertension (Batzdorf, 1976), which is a major factor in morbidity when a lumbar puncture is performed injudiciously. On theoretical and recent experimental grounds, corticosteroids — the principal pharmacological agents used in the management of cerebral oedema of non-infectious origin — seem to hinder sterilisation and localisation of a cerebritic process (Quartey et al., 1976); we therefore recommend the use of osmotic agents such as mannitol or urea. Definitive therapy includes surgical drainage and/or excision of the abscess, and abolition of the intra- or extra-cranial source of infection.

3. Epidural Abscess

Spinal epidural abscess may occur secondary to bacteraemic seeding from a remote pyogenic focus, septicaemia, or direct extension from vertebral osteomyelitis. Unless radiographs or radionuclide scans demonstrate osteomyelitis or a paraspinous collection of pus, laboratory studies other than blood culture and Gram stain of pus may be of relatively little help in defining the process.

The most common causative organism in most series has been *S. aureus* (Baker, 1971; Baker et al., 1975); unless other forms such as Gram-negative bacilli are seen on smear, the obtaining of appropriate cultures should be followed immediately by administration of a parenteral antistaphylococcal penicillin (e.g. cloxacillin), with subsequent therapy being guided by the results of cultures and susceptibility testing. Rapid assessment and antibiotic therapy should be followed by surgical exploration and drainage as soon as the patient is stable. Appropriate antibiotic therapy should be continued for no less than two weeks, and in the presence of vertebral osteomyelitis, probably for 4 to 6 weeks.

4. Subdural Empyema

Subdural effusions are common during the course of acute bacterial meningitis, though uncommonly manifest. If a persistent effusion remains infected and becomes confined or loculated, empyema results and may be recognised because of persisting or secondary fever, lateralising neurological signs, or elevated intracranial pressure. When empyema is associated with sinusitis, days or weeks of non-specific symptoms may be followed by sudden neurological deterioration (Kaufman et al., 1975; Leading Article, 1976). Empyema may also follow neurosurgical infection.

As with brain abscess, lumbar puncture may be dangerous in the presence of subdural empyema, with a high risk of transtentorial herniation of the brain (Kaufman et al., 1975). Inasmuch as the CSF is not diagnostic in this condition, its study may be deferred pending specific diagnostic studies such as cerebral angiography, radionuclide scanning (Gilday, 1974), or computerised axial tomography (Zimmerman et al., 1976).

4.1 Pathogenic Organisms

The microbiology of subdural empyema reflects the antecedent or associated infection. Post-meningitic empyema may contain the same organism initially isolated from lumbar CSF; those associated with sinusitis frequently contain anaerobes (Yoshikawa et al., 1976).

Table II. Summary of the treatment of bacterial infections of the central nervous system in infants and children

---

1. *Neonatal meningitis*
    a) Initiate treatment with IV ampicillin plus either gentamicin or kanamycin, pending results of cultures.
    b) Revise therapy as guided by testing of patient's isolate.
    c) Use penicillin G for pneumococcal and streptococcal meningitis; antistaphylococcal penicillin (e.g. cloxacillin) for staphylococcal meningitis.
    d) Monitor CSF to gauge progress.
    e) Examine ventricular fluid if progress is poor or cultures remain positive; instill gentamicin at time of ventricular puncture.
    f) Continue therapy for 2 weeks after first negative CSF culture.

2. *Purulent meningitis of childhood*
    a) Initiate treatment with IV ampicillin (400mg/kg/day), pending results of culture.
    b) Add chloramphenicol (100mg/kg/day) if ampicillin resistant strains of *H. influenzae* suspected; discontinue if subsequently found to be ampicillin sensitive.
    c) Use penicillin G alone if pneumococcus or meningococcus isolated.
    d) Continue therapy until child clinically satisfactory and afebrile for 5 days.

3. *Tuberculous meningitis*
    a) Traditional regimen: isoniazid + PAS + streptomycin.
    b) Rifampicin may eventually supplant PAS and streptomycin.

4. *Brain abscess*
    a) Initiate treatment with high dose penicillin G IV.
    b) Add chloramphenicol if *B. fragilis* isolated or suspected.
    c) Control intracranial hypertension with osmotic agents (mannitol or urea).
    d) Treat intra- or extra-cranial source of infection + surgical drainage and/or excision of abscess.

5. *Epidural abscess*
    a) Initiate treatment with parenteral antistaphylococcal penicillin (e.g. cloxacillin).
    b) Modify therapy on basis of culture results.
    c) Surgical drainage as soon as patient stable.

6. *Subdural empyema*
    a) Surgical drainage with bacteriological studies.
    b) Select antibiotic on basis of Gram stain of pus.
    c) Use chloramphenicol if small Gram-negative rods present (may be *Bacteroides* spp. or *Haemophilus* spp). Substitute ampicillin if isolate subsequently found to be sensitive by laboratory methods.
    d) Antistaphylococcal penicillin (e.g. cloxacillin) if Gram-positive cocci present.
    e) Treat infected sinuses, etc.

7. *CSF shunt infections*
    a) Culture ventricular fluid and blood.
    b) Initiate treatment with high dose penicillin G IV.
    c) Monitor CSF and serum levels of drug.
    d) Add intraventricular gentamicin (1 to 4mg), 12-hourly if necessary.
    e) Remove and replace shunt if antibiotic therapy fails.

4.2 Treatment

Treatment includes appropriate antibiotic therapy coupled with decompression and drainage. Initially, antibiotics may be selected on the basis of the Gram stain of pus obtained via subdural taps. Small Gram-negative rods may be *Bacteroides* spp., or *Haemophilus* spp., and against these organisms chloramphenicol remains the drug of choice in intracranial infections; ampicillin may be substituted for chloramphenicol if the isolate is subsequently found to be sensitive by laboratory methods. Clumps of Gram-positive cocci may represent staphylococci, for which an antistaphylococcal penicillin (e.g. cloxacillin) should be chosen. The remainder of the usual organisms, other than those found in wound infections, are penicillin sensitive.

Attention should also be paid to infected sinuses, etc., which should be drained as early as possible.

5. Cerebrospinal Fluid Shunt Infections

CSF shunts have proven a great advance in the management of hydrocephalus. Apart from their need for revision due to blockage or to linear growth of the child, the major cause of morbidity associated with their use is infection.

5.1 Pathogenic Organisms

The most common organism colonising shunts is the ordinarily saprophytic coagulase-negative *Staphylococcus epidermidis* (formerly called *S. albus)*, presumably introduced during surgical implantation of the shunt. *S. aureus* and a miscellany of other organisms are found much less frequently (Schoenbaum et al., 1975; Shurtleff et al., 1974).

Shunt infection must be considered in the differential diagnosis of any patient who presents with fever, malaise, shunt malfunction, or signs of increasing intracranial pressure, etc. Specific findings may include erythema over the subcutaneous tunnel of the shunt tubing, evidence of chronic bacteraemia such as splenomegaly and anaemia, or urinary abnormalities consistent with shunt nephritis (Rames et al., 1970). Examination and culture of the ventricular fluid is very important; ventricular CSF is most easily and atraumatically obtained if the shunt appliance incorporates a subcutaneous reservoir (Myers and Schoenbaum, 1975). The presence of *S. epidermidis* in the CSF and blood is diagnostic.

5.2 Treatment

The definitive treatment for a shunt which remains infected despite an adequate trial of antibiotic therapy, is complete removal and replacement of the apparatus.

However, non-operative management of infection may be successful and may be advocated as initial therapy (Idriss and Sisk, 1974; McLaurin, 1973; Shurtleff et al., 1974). *S. epidermidis* exhibits variable patterns of antibiotic resistance, and a blood or CSF isolate should be studied carefully. A penicillinase negative *S. epidermidis* with a low MIC and MBC (minimum inhibitory and bactericidal concentrations) of penicillin may be safely treated with high dose penicillin G, with monitoring of serum and CSF levels of drug or of inhibitory and killing power against the offending organism. Because of the relatively minor effect of this infection on the meninges and apparently on the functional blood-brain barrier, adequate concentrations of drug may not be attainable in the CSF. A number of workers have therefore resorted to intraventricular instillation, through the shunt reservoir if present; however, ventricular concentrations of drug fall rapidly as the CSF drains out through the shunt, and doses may have to be given every 12 hours (McLaurin, 1973). Depending on the size of the patient's CSF space, intraventricular doses of antibiotics proposed include: gentamicin 1 to 4mg; methicillin or cephalothin 25 to 50mg (McLaurin, 1973); we have found gentamicin safe and effective.

The optimum duration of intraventricular and systemic therapy, and prospective criteria of therapeutic success of non-operative management, have yet to be determined.

References

Ahronheim, G.A.: *Haemophilus influenzae* type b: Lack of in-vitro antagonism between penicillins and chloramphenicol. Pediatric Research 9: 337, 1975.

Ahronheim, G.A. and Marks, M.I.: Recurrent meningitis due to a pneumococcus type 23 relatively resistant to penicillin: Failure of penicillin prophylaxis and therapy. Paper presented to the Royal College of Physicians of Canada, Toronto, 1977.

American Academy of Pediatrics (Committee on Infectious Disease): Current status of ampicillin-resistant *Hemophilus influenzae* type b. Pediatrics 57: 417 (1976).

Baker, A.S.; Ojemann, R.G.; Swartz, M.N. and Richardson, E.P.: Spinal epidural abscess. New England Journal of Medicine 293: 463-468 (1975).

Baker, C.J.: Primary spinal epidural abscess. American Journal of Diseases of Children 339 (1971).

Baker, C.J.; Barrett, F.F.; Gordon, R.C. and Yow, M.D.: Suppurative meningitis due to streptococci of Lancefield Group B. A study of 33 infants. Journal of Pediatrics 82: 724-729 (1973).

Barton, L.L.; Feigin, R.D. and Lins, R.: Group B beta-hemolytic streptococcal meningitis in infants. Journal of Pediatrics 82: 719-723 (1973).

Batzdorf, U.: The management of cerebral edema in pediatric practice. Pediatrics 58: 78-87 (1976).

Bell, W.E. and McCormick, W.F.: in Neurologic Infections in Children (Saunders, Philadelphia 1975).

Black, P.; Graybill, J.R. and Charache, P.: Penetration of brain abscess by systemically administered antibiotics. Journal of Neurosurgery 38: 705-709 (1973).

Catlin, B.W.: Iodometric detection of *Haemophilus influenzae* beta-lactamase: Rapid presumptive test for ampicillin resistance. Antimicrobial Agents and Chemotherapy 7: 265-270 (1975).

DuPont, H.L.; Hornick, R.B.; Weiss, C.F.; Snyder, M.J. and Woodward, T.E.: Evaluation of chloramphenicol acid succinate therapy of induced typhoid fever and Rocky Mountain spotted fever. New England Journal of Medicine 282: 53-57 (1970).

Eickhoff, T.C. and Marks, M.I.: Carbenicillin in therapy of systemic infections due to *Pseudomonas*. Journal of Infectious Diseases 122 (Suppl.): S84-S86 (1970).

Escamilla, J.: Susceptibility of *Haemophilus influenzae* to ampicillin as determined by use of a modified, one-minute beta-lactamase test. Antimicrobial Agents and Chemotherapy 9: 196-198 (1976).

Fallon, R.J.: *Haemophilus influenzae* meningitis. Journal of Antimicrobial Chemotherapy 2: 3-5, 1976.

Fischbein, C.A.; Rosenthal, A.; Fischer, E.G.; Nadas, A.S. and Welch, K.: Risk factors for brain abscess in patients with congenital heart disease. American Journal of Cardiology 34: 97-102 (1974).

Fisher, L.S.; Chow, A.W.; Yoshikawa, T.T. and Guze, L.B.: Cephalothin and cephaloridine therapy for bacterial meningitis. Annals of Internal Medicine 82: 689-693 (1975).

Frederick, J. and Braude, A.I.: Anaerobic infection of the paranasal sinuses. New England Journal of Medicine 290: 135-137 (1974).

Gaman, W.; Cates, C.; Snelling, C.F.T.; Lank, B. and Ronald, A.R.: Emergence of gentamicin- and carbenicillin-resistant *Pseudomonas aeruginosa* in a hospital environment. Antimicrobial Agents and Chemotherapy 9: 474-480 (1976).

Gilday, D.: Various radionuclide patterns of cerebral inflammation in infants and children. American Journal of Roentgenology, Radium Therapy and Nuclear Medicine 120: 247-253 (1974).

Goldacre, M.J.: Acute bacterial meningitis in childhood. Incidence and mortality in a defined population. Lancet 1: 28 (1976).

Greene, B.M.; Thomas, F.E. and Alford, R.H.: Trimethoprim-sulfamethoxazole and brain abscess. Annals of Internal Medicine 82: 812-813 (1975).

Hansman, D.: Type distribution and antibiotic sensitivity of *Diplococcus pneumoniae:* A 5-year study in Sydney. Medical Journal of Australia 2: 436-440 (1974).

Hawley, H.B. and Gump, D.W.: Vancomycin therapy of bacterial meningitis. American Journal of Diseases of Children 126: 261-264 (1973).

Hewitt, W.L. and Winters, R.E.: The current status of parenteral carbenicillin. Journal of Infectious Diseases 127 (Suppl.): S120-S129 (1973).

Heineman, H.S. and Braude, A.I.: Anaerobic infection of the brain. American Journal of Medicine 35: 682-697 (1963).

Hollifield, J.W.; Kaiser, A.B. and McGee, Z.A.: Gram-negative bacillary meningitis therapy. Polyradiculitis following intralumbar aminoglycoside administration. Journal of the American Medical Association 236: 1264-1266 (1976).

Howard, J.B. and McCracken, G.H.: Reappraisal of kanamycin usage in neonates. Journal of Pediatrics 86: 949-956 (1975a).

Howard, J.B. and McCracken, G.H.: Pharmacological evaluation of amikacin in neonates. Antimicrobial Agents and Chemotherapy 8: 86-90 (1975b).

Idriss, Z.H. and Sisk, M.A.: Medical treatment of infected cerebrospinal fluid shunts. Lebanese Medical Journal 27: 205-208 (1974).

Idriss, Z.H.; Sinno, A.A. and Kronfol, N.M.: Tuberculous meningitis in childhood. American Journal of Diseases of Children 130: 364-367 (1976).

Ingham, H.R.; Selkon, J.B. and Roxby, C.M.: Bacteriological study of otogenic cerebral abscesses: Chemotherapeutic role of metronidazole. British Medical Journal 2: 991-993 (1977).

Jorgensen, J.G. and Lee, J.C.: Microdilution technique for antimicrobial susceptibility testing of *Haemophilus influenzae*. Antimicrobial Agents and Chemotherapy 8: 610-611 (1975).

Kaiser, A.B. and McGee, Z.A.: Aminoglycoside therapy of Gram-negative bacillary meningitis. New England Journal of Medicine 293: 1215-1220 (1975).

Kannan, M.M.; Dalton, H.P. and Escobar, M.R.: Tobramycin in the neonatal period. Virginia Medical Monthly 100: 1030-1034 (1973).

Kaplan, J.M.; McCracken, G.H.; Thomas, M.L.; Horton, L.J. and Davis, N.: Clinical pharmacology of tobramycin in newborns. American Journal of Diseases of Children 125: 656-660 (1973).

Katz, S.L.: Ampicillin-resistant *Hemophilus influenzae* type b: A status report. Pediatrics 55: 6-8 (1975).

Kaufman, D.M.; Miller, M.H. and Steigbigel, N.H.: Subdural empyema: Analysis of 17 recent cases and review of the literature. Medicine 54: 485-498 (1975).

Leading Article: Nova et vetera. Lancet 1: 676-677 (1976).

McCracken, G.H.: Pharmacological basis for antimicrobial therapy in newborn infants. American Journal of Diseases of Children 128: 407-419 (1974).

McCracken, G.H.: Editorial comment. Journal of Pediatrics 89: 203-204 (1976).

McCracken, G.H. and Eichenwald, H.F.: Antimicrobial therapy: Therapeutic recommendations and a review of newer drugs. Journal of Pediatrics 85: 297-312 and 451-456 (1974).

McCracken, G.H. and Mize, S.G.: A controlled study of intrathecal antibiotic therapy in Gram-negative enteric meningitis of infancy. Journal of Pediatrics 89: 66-72 (1976).

McCracken, G.H. and Threlkeld, N.: Kanamycin dosage in newborn infants. Journal of Pediatrics 89: 313-314 (1976).

McLaurin, R.L.: Infected cerebrospinal fluid shunts. Surgical Neurology 1: 191-195 (1973).

Marks, M.I.: In vitro antibacterial activity of amikacin, a new aminoglycoside, against clinical bacterial isolates from children. Journal of Clinical Pharmacology 15: 246-251 (1975).

Marks, M.I. and Weinmaster, G.: Influences of media and inocula on the in vitro susceptibility of *Haemophilus influenzae* to co-trimoxazole, ampicillin, penicillin, and chloramphenicol. Antimicrobial Agents and Chemotherapy 8: 657-663 (1975).

Mathies, A.W.: Penicillins in the treatment of bacterial meningitis. Journal of the Royal College of Physicians (London) 6: 139-146 (1972).

Myers, M.G. and Schoenbaum, S.C.: Shunt fluid aspiration. An adjunct in the diagnosis of cerebrospinal fluid shunt infection. American Journal of Diseases of Children 129: 220-222 (1975).

Naraqi, S.; Kirkpatrick, G.P. and Kabins, S.: Relapsing pneumococcal meningitis: Isolation of an organism with decreased susceptibility to penicillin G. Journal of Pediatrics 85: 671-673 (1974).

Nelson, J.D. and McCracken, G.H.: Clinical pharmacology of carbenicillin and gentamicin in the neonate and comparative efficacy with ampicillin and gentamicin. Pediatrics 52: 802-812 (1973).

Quartey, G.E.C.; Johnston, J.A. and Rodzilsky, B.: Decadron in the treatment of cerebral abscess: An experimental study. Journal of Neurosurgery 45: 301-310 (1976).

Rames, L.; Wise, B.; Goodman, J.R. and Piel, C.F.: Renal disease with *Staphylococcus albus* bacteremia. Journal of the American Medical Association 212: 1671-1677 (1970).

Salmon, J.H.: Ventriculitis complicating meningitis. American Journal of Diseases of Children 124: 35-40 (1972).

Schoenbaum, S.C.; Gardner, P. and Shillito, J.: Infections of cerebrospinal fluid shunts: Epidemiology, clinical manifestations and therapy. Journal of Infectious Diseases 131: 543-552 (1975).

Shurtleff, D.B.; Foltz, E.L.; Weeks, R.D. and Loeser, J.: Therapy of *Staphylococcus epidermidis:* Infections associated with cerebrospinal fluid shunts. Pediatrics 53: 55-62 (1974).

Sifontes, J.E.: Rifampin in tuberculous meningitis. Journal of Pediatrics 87: 1015-1017 (1975).

Smith, A.L.: Tuberculous meningitis in childhood. Medical Journal of Australia 1: 57-60 (1975).

Smith, A.L.: Current concepts: Antibiotics and invasive *Haemophilus influenzae.* New England Journal of Medicine 294: 1329-1331 (1976).

Smith, D.H.; Ingram, D.L.; Smith, A.L.; Gilles, F. and Bresnan, M.J.: Bacterial meningitis: A symposium. Pediatrics 52: 586-600 (1973).

Steiner, P. and Portugaleza, C.: Tuberculous meningitis in children. American Review of Respiratory Disease 107: 22-29 (1973).

Sumaya, C.V.; Simek, M.; Smith, M.H.D.; Ferriss, G.S. and Rubin, W.: Tuberculous meningitis in children during the isoniazid era. Journal of Pediatrics 87: 43-49 (1975).

Swartz, M.N. and Dodge, P.R.: Bacterial meningitis: A review of selected aspects. New England Journal of Medicine 272: 725-731, 779-787, 842-848, 898-902, 954-960 and 1003-1010 (1965).

Thornsberry, C. and Kirven, L.A.: Ampicillin susceptibility of *Haemophilus influenza*. Antimicrobial Agents and Chemotherapy 6: 620-624 (1974a).

Thornsberry, C. and Kirven, L.A.: Ampicillin-resistance in *Haemophilus influenzae* as determined by a rapid test for beta-lactamase production. Antimicrobial Agents and Chemotherapy 6: 653-654 (1974b).

Visudhiphan, P. and Chiemchanya, S.: Evaluation of rifampicin in the treatment of tuberculous meningitis in children. Journal of Pediatrics 87: 983-986 (1975).

Yoshikawa, T.T.; Chow, A.W. and Guze, L.B.: Role of anaerobic bacteria in subdural empyema. American Journal of Medicine 58: 99-104 (1976).

Yoshikawa, T.T. and Goodman, S.J.: Brain abscess. Western Journal of Medicine 121: 207-219 (1974).

Yow, M.D.; Baker, C.J.; Barrett, F.F. and Ortigoza, C.O.: Initial antibiotic management of bacterial meningitis (selection in relationship to age). Medicine 52: 305-308 (1973).

Zimmerman, R.A.; Patel, S. and Bilaniuk, L.T.: Demonstration of purulent bacterial intracranial infections by computed tomography. American Journal of Roentgenology 127: 155-165 (1976).

Chapter IV

Genitourinary Infections

M.I. Marks

Acute and chronic urinary tract infections are common in children. In the newborn period, the pathogenesis is usually haematogenous and males are more frequently infected than females. A second incidence peak occurs in preschool age children where the pathogenesis involves faecal contamination and ascending infection. Females predominate in this group as well as in school age and sexually active children with urinary infections. *Escherichia coli* is the major bacterial pathogen at all ages.

These infections, as well as specific infectious syndromes of the urethra and bladder, are discussed in this chapter.

1. Urethritis

1.1 Pathogenesis

Inflammation of the urethra in children has many aetiologies. Non-infectious causes such as trauma, bubble bath detergents and other irritants are more common in young children, while infectious urethritis due to *N. gonorrhoeae* or other microorganisms such as *Chlamydia trachomatis* and *Ureaplasma urealyticum* ('non-gonococcal or post-gonococcal' urethritis) [Bowie et al., 1976; Holmes et al., 1975] are more common in sexually active adolescents. Other infectious causes of urethritis include *Candida albicans*, *Trichomonas vaginalis*, *Mima polymorpha*, *Herpes simplex* type 2, *Enterobius vermicularis* and syphilis. Enteric bacteria and parasites may also cause acute urethritis secondary to faecal contamination, particularly in young children.

1.2 Clinical Features

The clinical picture of gonorrhoea is one of acute onset of dysuria and exudative urethritis with a profuse yellow discharge. This usually occurs 2 to 8 days after sexual intercourse. The condition may also be asymptomatic in both males and females. Leucorrhoea may be the most prominent sign in girls and dysuria may be absent. Arthritis, asymptomatic pyuria, skin lesions and balanitis may be occasional presenting signs as well. Newborns are at risk of developing conjunctivitis due to exposure to the gonococcus in the mother's birth canal.

The spread of gonorrhoea is predominantly sexual in the adolescent and even in prepubescent children, although non-venereal contact has been demonstrated to be responsible in several cases (Shore and Winkelstein, 1971).

Non-gonococcal urethritis is characterised by a longer incubation period (5 to 14 days) after sexual intercourse and has a scanty, often clear, discharge. The usual causes of this condition are *Chlamydia trachomatis* (Bowie et al., 1976) and *Ureaplasma urealyticum* (Holmes et al., 1975). These infections account for approximately 80% of non-gonococcal urethritis in sexually active patients.

1.3 Diagnosis

Gram stain of the urethral discharge in the male, and cultures in both male and female (urethral cultures in adolescent boys and girls; urethral, endocervical and rectal cultures in adolescent females and vaginal cultures in prepubescent females) are necessary to diagnose gonorrhoea and to differentiate this condition from non-gonococcal urethritis (Kellogg et al., 1976).

1.4 Treatment

1.4.1 Gonococcal Urethritis

The treatment of gonococcal urethritis has been studied in children and several regimens are equally effective (Nelson et al., 1976). Single dose therapy employing procaine penicillin 100,000u/kg IM (maximum 4.8 mega u) or amoxycillin 50mg/kg orally (maximum 3.5g) have been used; each of these is immediately preceded by probenecid 25mg/kg orally (maximum 1g) [Kellogg et al., 1976]. Cure rates of over 90% can be expected with these regimens. Repeat urethral cultures are indicated 48 hours after institution of therapy if symptoms are not considerably improved and 1 week after therapy in all patients. Both of these are necessary to exclude penicillinase producing bacteria (Wilkinson et al., 1976) and to detect relapses and recurrences.

Penicillin sensitive individuals and those with penicillin resistant gonococci should be treated with either spectinomycin 2g IM (adult dose) or tetracycline 500mg orally 4 times a day for 4 days (adult dose) [Karney et al., 1977]. Erythromycin and co-trimoxazole are less adequate therapy for gonococcal urethritis (Karney et al., 1977). All cases need careful follow-up, serological tests for syphilis at the time of diagnosis and 2 to 3 months thereafter, and careful educational, hygienic and psychosocial counselling. Counselling is particularly important in prepubescent children with gonorrhoea. Intervention by social agencies is occasionally necessary.

Non-urethral gonorrhoea infections (i.e. pharyngitis, bacteraemia, arthritis, salpingitis and proctitis) should be treated by more prolonged and intensive antibiotic therapy. The ubiquitous nature of gonorrhoea and its growing worldwide prevalence, the development of antibiotic resistance and complications pursuant to repeated courses of urethritis (e.g. urethral stricture, pelvic inflammatory disease, salpingitis and infertility) warrant careful attention to diagnosis and therapy in this condition.

1.4.2 Non-gonococcal Urethritis and Post-gonococcal Urethritis

These conditions are most effectively treated by a 2 to 3 week course of tetracycline 500mg 4 times a day (adult dose). Careful follow-up to rule out gonorrhoea and syphilis as well as therapy of contacts is important for these conditions, as it is for gonorrhoea and syphilis.

1.4.3 Other Forms of Infectious Urethritis

Other causes of infectious urethritis include *Trichomonas vaginalis* which is best treated with metronidazole or tinidazole. Again, contacts should be treated simultaneously.

Staphylococci, streptococci and occasionally faecal contaminants may be causative organisms in sudden-onset urethritis in younger children. These should be treated with appropriate short term (5 to 7 days) antibiotic therapy based on culture and sensitivity data in each case.

Candida albicans infections can be treated with local applications of nystatin. Infections due to *Enterobius vermicularis* (pinworms) are best treated with oral viprynium (pyrvinium) pamoate (5mg/kg orally) or pyrantel pamoate (10mg/kg orally) administered as a single dose to all family members and repeated in two weeks.

1.4.4 Non-infectious Urethritis

Non-infectious causes of urethritis such as detergents, trauma, foreign bodies, usually depend on other diagnostic criteria and therapy should be directed at removing the offending cause and proper counselling.

2. Cystitis

2.1 Pathogenesis

Most (approximately 80%) cases of cystitis occur in females and are secondary to infection with *Escherichia coli* (Welch et al., 1976). Younger children may commonly have faecal contamination and infection with enteric bacteria, while in older children, trauma, masturbation and retrograde milking of the urethra during sexual intercourse may facilitate the introduction of bacteria into the bladder and cause cystitis. The shorter female urethra, increased retrograde contamination, and oestrogens have been postulated as important factors in females (Harle et al., 1975). The antibacterial effect of prostatic secretions in males may partly explain their resistance to bacterial cystitis (Fair and Wehner, 1971).

Cystitis often accompanies urethritis and/or pyelonephritis.

2.2 Clinical Features

Clinical features of cystitis include abrupt onset of dysuria, suprapubic pain, frequency, urgency and occasionally haematuria. Investigators have used these clinical criteria plus the absence of back or renal pain, mild temperature (elevations to less than 38.5°C) and the presence of significant bacteriuria to define bacterial cystitis (Kaijser, 1973).

2.2.1 Asymptomatic Bacteriuria

Asymptomatic bacteriuria is a common problem which will be discussed in more detail below (section 3.2). Approximately half of these patients can be clearly defined as having only cystitis by investigational techniques (Lindberg et al., 1975). Commercial kits are available for screening normal children for the presence of asymptomatic bacteriuria (Barry et al., 1975; Gillenwater et al., 1976). These are of two types; one depends on microbiological growth and the other on chemical changes due to bacterial metabolism. Of the two, the microbiological tests seem to be more reliable, as the numbers of false positives and false negatives encountered in the chemical tests may be as high as 10 and 15%, respectively (Gillenwater et al., 1976). Microbiological screening tests are useful, but should only be used in normal healthy populations and as a guideline to more careful laboratory microbiology. The latter is necessary to clearly identify the organisms involved and to quantitate the infection to allow for statistical confidence in the diagnosis as outlined below (section 2.5.3). *In vitro* susceptibility tests also depend on careful isolation of bacteria in pure culture.

2.2.2 Viral Cystitis

Viral cystitis usually presents with sudden onset of painful haematuria and the bacterial culture of the urine is sterile. Adenovirus 11 and, rarely, adenovirus 21 are causes of this syndrome and males are more frequently affected than females, the ratio being approximately 3:1 (Numazaki et al., 1973).

2.3 Predisposing Factors

Factors predisposing to the development of cystitis include congenital and acquired obstructions. Included in the former category are patients with obstruction of the bladder outlet, urethra and meatus. This was formerly considered to be a common syndrome; however, many of the radiographic findings including reflux and abnormal micturition have been subsequently shown to be variations in normal excretory patterns (Shopfner et al., 1970). They may also be related to persisting inflammation at the time of radiographic examination (Barry et al., 1975).

Neuromuscular disorders such as meningomyelocele may also lead to neurogenic bladder. Here again, abnormalities in urination leading to obstruction and stasis are conditions predisposing to the development of cystitis. Occasional patients with megacolon due to Hirschsprung's disease may have congenital and acquired obstruction due to faecal impaction as a basis for their cystitis.

Repeated infections, trauma, indwelling urethral catheters and post-surgical conditions also predispose the host to secondary cystitis.

2.4 Other Causes of Cystitis

Rare causes of infectious cystitis include tuberculosis, schistosomiasis and other parasitic infestations including toxocariasis, filariasis and *Enterobius vermicularis*. These conditions can lead to a granulomatous appearance of the bladder, or may be associated with eosinophilia in the case of parasitic infestations. Rarely, gas-forming micro-organisms including bacteria and fungi may give rise to emphysematous cystitis and clinical symptoms of pneumaturia (Marks, 1971).

Occasionally, neuropsychiatric disorders may cause symptoms of cystitis such as frequency, urgency, daytime dribbling, nocturnal enuresis and abdominal pain (Welch et al., 1976). Exclusion of neuropsychiatric pathology is recommended before making less well defined diagnoses such as interstitial cystitis or small bladder syndromes (Geist and Antolak, 1969). The latter conditions have been described in the urological literature to explain certain children with enuresis and lower abdominal symptoms compatible with cystitis. They are poorly defined histopathologically and clinically, and surgical intervention including cystoscopy is rarely indicated,

2.5 Diagnosis

A normal urinalysis and a negative bacterial culture are useful in excluding cystitis.

2.5.1 Collection of Urine

False positive results are often due to inappropriate urine collection such as specimens obtained by adhesive bag, those not cultured or refrigerated immediately after collection, or obtained without careful preparation and midstream technique (particularly in patients who have gastroenteritis, poor hygiene or who are menstruating, etc.) [Barry et al., 1975; Pryles and Lustik, 1971]. In ill patients with pronounced signs of acute bacterial cystitis, suprapubic bladder aspiration is rapid, safe and reliable for obtaining urine for analysis and culture (Barry et al., 1975; Pryles and Lustik, 1971). Therapy may then be instituted immediately. Otherwise, a clean-catch midstream urine sample should be used.

Urethral catheterisation may be traumatic, may introduce infection into the bladder and may make quantitative bacteriology difficult to interpret. If urine is obtained from an indwelling intraurethral catheter, it should be obtained via the direct aspiration from the tubing.

2.5.2 Urinalysis

Urinalysis should be performed in a standardised manner. Approximately 5 ml of urine is centrifuged at 3000 rpm for 3 minutes and examined by light microscopy. Abundant bacteria (too numerous to count) in an unstained preparation of the sediment from this sample can be correlated with the presence of significant bacteriuria in over 90 % of cases. The presence of bacteria in a Gram stain of uncentrifuged urine can also be correlated with significant bacteriuria in over 95 % of cases. Visualisation of more than 5 white blood cells per high power field correlates with significant bacteriuria in approximately 50 % of cases. Pyuria may also be seen in states of extreme dehydration, after trauma, with a foreign body or chemical irritation, and after oral polio vaccine administration (Pryles and Lustik, 1971).

2.5.3 Urine Culture

The presence of more than 100,000 colonies/ml of a single bacterial type in pure growth from a urine culture obtained by the clean-catch technique, correlates with the presence of true urinary tract infection in 80 % of cases; two consecutive cultures with these results offers 95 % accuracy, and 3 or more cultures close to 100 % accuracy (Barry et al., 1975). Occasionally, urine counts between 10,000 and 100,000/ml may be due to increased excretion rates due to fluid diuresis, an extremely low pH, bacteriostatic substances in the urine, or infection due to fastidious organisms (Pryles and Lustik, 1971). Rarely, intermittent obstruction may also give rise to confusing results.

Any pathogenic bacteria isolated from a suprapubic bladder aspiration is considered significant.

2.6 Treatment

2.6.1 Curative Therapy

Treatment of bacterial cystitis in children can be effectively carried out by use of a variety of antibacterial drugs which are excreted by the kidneys. These drugs are highly concentrated in the urine so that even oral penicillin G which attains only modest plasma levels can be used to treat some infections (Hulbert, 1972). However, other antibacterials (e.g. sulphonamides, ampicillin/amoxycillin, co-trimoxazole or nitrofurantoin) are preferred, because they are better distributed in the tissues of the urinary tract and relatively more resistant to bacterial β-lactamases. A two week course of therapy should be adequate in the majority of cases. Shorter durations of therapy are probably appropriate when the patient clearly has cystitis associated with urethritis. Recently, single dose therapy with amoxycillin (100mg/kg) and co-trimoxazole (0.72 to 1.44g) has been shown to be as effective as 5 to 7-day regimens of the same drugs in children with cystitis (Bailey and Abbott, 1977, 1978). However, experience with these regimens is limited, and frequently the difficulty of differentiating lower from upper urinary tract disease justifies a two week treatment course with x-ray examination (IVP) 6 weeks after eradication of the infection.

Patients with urinary tract infections should be recultured 48 to 72 hours after institution of therapy and 48 hours after completion of therapy. This is to ensure that bacteriological sterilisation of the urine during therapy correlates with clinical improvement, as well as to ensure complete eradication of the bacterial infection in the patient after therapy. Further follow-up cultures at 2 weeks, 3 months and 6 monthly intervals thereafter for 2 years, are indicated to exclude asymptomatic recurrences and as a guide to the need for long term therapy (Kunin, 1976).

Rarely, cystoscopy is indicated in patients with cystitis where foreign bodies, trauma or unusual parasitic infestations are suspected.

2.6.2 Prophylactic Therapy

The presence of one or more recurrences and/or the presence of congenital or acquired obstructions and abnormal urinary tract drainage are indications for long term chemoprophylaxis. Drugs such as co-trimoxazole, sulphonamides, nitrofurantoin, or hexamine (methenamine) mandelate or hippurate are all useful (Gerstein et al., 1968;

Kunin, 1976; Welch et al., 1976), although recent evidence suggests that hexamine preparations may not be as effective as the other drugs (Vainrub and Musher, 1977). Patient compliance is essential as are careful follow-up cultures and clinical examinations. Recurrences are rare during chemoprophylaxis but common after prophylaxis is stopped. The condition may disappear during adolescence or young adulthood or may reappear during sexual activity or during pregnancy in the form of asymptomatic bacteriuria.

2.7 Prognosis

The long term prognosis is excellent as progressive radiological findings of pyelonephritis are rare, as is the development of hypertension and loss of renal function (Dodge et al., 1974; Savage et al., 1975; Welch et al., 1976).

3. Upper Urinary Tract Infection

Since it is often impossible to clearly define the specific location of inflammation in urinary tract infection with any degree of confidence, many features of the pathogenesis, diagnosis and treatment are common to both upper and lower urinary tract infections. The reader is therefore referred to the previous section on cystitis as well for a more complete review of these subjects.

Pyelonephritis can be defined histopathologically as a collection of polymorphonuclear leucocytes, necrosis of renal epithelial cells, varying degrees of interstitial oedema, and debris. Bacterial antigens and micro-abscesses may or may not be present. Occasionally chronic suppurative renal infections can be granulomatous in appearance (Klugo et al., 1977). There is a loss of concentrating ability with bacterial infection of the kidney. There may also be a reversible decrease in glomerular filtration and excretion in patients with underlying obstructive uropathy.

3.1 Pathogenesis

The major causative bacteria of pyelonephritis in all age groups is *E. coli*, accounting for over 90 % of first urinary tract infections in girls and approximately 80 % of infections in newborns and young infants (Kunin, 1975; Kaijser et al., 1977). *E. coli* is detected in 60 to 65 % of first infections in boys and Proteus is a frequent second offender (Hallett et al., 1976). Several enteric bacteria, staphylococci, and occasionally *Candida albicans* and other fungi, may also be responsible for urinary tract infection in patients with chronic recurrent disease, and in those with underlying structural abnormalities and other predisposing host factors.

Table I. Summary of the treatment of common genitourinary infections in infants and children

---

1. *Urethritis*
   a) Gram stain of urethral discharge (males) and cultures necessary to distinguish gonorrhoea from non-gonococcal and other forms of urethritis.
   b) *Gonococcal urethritis:* treat with single-dose procaine penicillin (100,000u/kg IM) or amoxycillin (50mg/kg po), preceded by probenecid (25mg/kg po). If penicillin sensitive or resistant gonococcus present, give spectinomycin (2g IM — adult dose) or tetracycline (500mg qid x 4 days — adult dose).
   c) *Non-gonococcal urethritis:* treat with tetracycline (500mg qid x 2 to 3 weeks — adult dose).
   d) *Trichomoniasis:* treat with metronidazole or tinidazole.
   e) Careful medical and educational follow-up necessary in all patients and contacts. Syphilis should be ruled out.

2. *Cystitis*
   a) Confirm diagnosis with urinalysis and clean-catch or suprapubic bacterial culture of urine.
   b) *Curative therapy:* Give 2-week course of a sulphonamide, ampicillin/amoxycillin, co-trimoxazole or nitrofurantoin.
   c) Re-culture urine 48 to 72 hours after starting therapy and 48 hours after completion (to confirm urine sterile).
   d) Further follow-up cultures at 2 weeks, 3 months and 6 months.
   e) *Prophylactic therapy* (necessary if one or more recurrences or urological abnormalities present): Give long-term therapy with nitrofurantoin, sulphonamides, co-trimoxazole or hexamine (methenamine).

3. *Pyelonephritis*
   a) Confirm diagnosis with clean-catch or suprapubic urine culture.
   b) Investigate and treat (if possible) urological abnormalities.
   c) *Curative therapy:* Give 2-week course of ampicillin/amoxycillin, co-trimoxazole or sulphafurazole (sulfisoxazole).
   d) Re-culture urine 48 hours after starting therapy.
   e) If necessary, modify treatment on basis of *in vitro* susceptibility testing; give aminoglycosides (e.g. gentamicin) if septicaemia present.
   f) *Prophylactic therapy* (necessary if frequent recurrences or urological abnormalities present): Give long term therapy with nitrofurantoin, co-trimoxazole, sulphonamides or hexamine (methenamine).

3.2 Clinical Features

Clinical features of upper urinary tract infections include fever, flank pain, costovertebral angle tenderness, chills, and occasionally nausea, vomiting and diarrhoea in young patients. Newborns may manifest urinary tract infection as colic or jaundice (Du, 1976). The spectrum of clinical presentations also includes asymptomatic bacteriuria.

Kunin (1976) has described the frequency of urinary infection in girls to be around 1% and 0.3% in boys. Approximately 10% of asymptomatic bacteriuria in girls can be localised to the kidney while an additional 40 % can be localised to the bladder; considerable overlap is present in the remaining patients (Lindberg et al., 1975). Pyelonephritis is rare in newborns occurring in approximately 1/1000 subjects; prematures and males are more frequently infected (Edelmann et al., 1973). The infection usually occurs by the haematogenous route in this age group and a history of maternal urinary tract infection during gestation is often present. Retrograde infection from faecal carriage sites is involved in older patients and in such cases girls are more frequently infected than boys.

Infections in boys are more commonly associated with underlying renal abnormalities which can be diagnosed radiographically. Several studies indicate the incidence of major structural abnormalities may be as high as 40 to 50 % in boys and 20 % in girls (Saxena et al., 1975). Preschool girls with clear evidence of urethritis and cystitis have a much lower frequency of genitourinary abnormalities.

3.3 Diagnosis

The diagnosis of pyelonephritis depends on the clinical signs mentioned above and a careful examination of the urine (see also section 2.5). The presence of white blood cell casts, although rare, is an important sign of renal involvement. A completely normal urinalysis may be present in early stages of infection or with intermittent or unilateral obstruction syndromes. Because of these considerations the urinalysis serves as a presumptive tool and should never be the only basis for the diagnosis of the urinary tract infection (Pryles and Lustik, 1971). Urine culture obtained by careful midstream clean-catch technique or by suprapubic aspiration is necessary to confirm the diagnosis (see section 2.5.3). Once having made a diagnosis of urinary tract infection, the clinician has a responsibility to ensure that careful radiological, microbiological and follow-up surveillance examinations are performed. The frequency of recurrences (40 % in the first year decreasing to 1 % in the sixth year) after the first urinary tract infection in children is so great that a six year follow-up is often recommended for pyelonephritis (Cohen, 1972).

3.4 Radiological Examination

Radiological examination should be performed approximately 6 weeks after cure in patients with a diagnosis of pyelonephritis to rule out structural abnormalities. Earlier radiological examination will describe reflux and residual urine as well as features of out-flow obstruction in as many as 50 % of the patients. At least one-half of these revert to normal on later examination (Forbes et al., 1969). Most of these abnormalities are not amenable to surgical therapy although the prognosis for recurrence may be more guarded in patients with persisting abnormalities. Many of these features are secondary to oedema and inflammatory reaction at the urethral uretero-vesical junction or in the bladder neck and urethra.

In situations where the clinical presentation (such as the persistence of severe colicky pain, resistance to treatment despite *in vitro* susceptibility, detection of a mass lesion in the abdomen or the presence of hypertension or renal functional impairment) suggests the presence of nephrolithiasis or other obstruction, earlier intravenous pyelography and retrograde cystourethrography may also be indicated. Cystoscopy, radioisotope scans, image-intensifying scans and voiding cystourethrograms are rarely indicated in patients with pyelonephritis.

3.5 Treatment

3.5.1 Curative Therapy

Escherichia coli pyelonephritis is usually treated with ampicillin/amoxycillin, co-trimoxazole or sulphafurazole (sulfisoxazole) in conventional therapeutic dosages (table II) for approximately 2 weeks. Follow-up culture 48 hours after institution of therapy will objectively supplement the clinical impression that the therapy is effective. If clinical signs are still present 72 hours after infection and/or the urine culture is still positive, *in vitro* susceptibility testing should be used as a guide to further chemotherapy. Hydration is a useful adjunct to antibiotic therapy.

Kanamycin, gentamicin, or tobramycin are extremely useful in the treatment of pyelonephritis associated with septicaemia and should be used in maximal doses because of the threat of the bacteraemia.

It should be remembered that the sulphonamides are most soluble and active in an alkaline pH and this may be important in hydropenic states. The penicillins and hexamine (methenamine) are generally more active in an acid pH while the activity of the aminoglycosides and erythromycin against Gram-negative bacteria is enhanced in an alkaline pH (Mou, 1962).

Infants and children rarely require analgesics during the treatment of urinary tract infection. If they do, aspirin or codeine may be used.

3.5.2 Prophylactic Therapy

The prophylaxis of chronic urinary tract infections depends on the cause. For example, neurogenic bladder infections can be minimised with urinary antiseptics and also with frequent emptying of the bladder by intermittent urethral catheterisation (Orikasa et al., 1976). The use of ileal conduits is no longer recommended because of the frequency of recurrent infections and obstruction (Middleton and Hendren, 1976). Colonic diversions and other drainage procedures are more useful but rarely indicated. These patients, plus those with underlying renal abnormalities that cannot

Table II. Guide to the use of antibacterial drugs in the treatment of paediatric urinary tract infections

Antibacterial drug	Dose and route	Side Effects
Amoxycillin	25 to 50mg/kg/day po divided q6h	Hypersensitivity-rash, urticaria, diarrhoea
Ampicillin	50 to 100mg/kg/day po or IV divided q6h	As for amoxycillin
Co-trimoxazole (trimethoprim + sulphamethoxazole in a 1:5 ratio)	25 to 50mg sulphamethoxazole/kg/day po divided q12h Inappropriate for newborns	Rash, nausea, vomiting Leucopenia, anaemia Haemolysis in G6PD deficiency
Gentamicin	*Infants less than 2kg:* 5mg/kg/day IV/IM divided q12 to 24h for first week, then 7.5mg/kg/day divided q12h *Infants more than 2kg:* 5 to 7.5mg/kg/day IV/IM divided q12h for first week, then q8h *Older children:* 5 to 6mg/kg/day IV/IM divided q8h	Ototoxic and possibly nephrotoxic Slow infusion necessary Dosages up to 7.5mg/kg/day may be used for short periods for severe infections Ototoxicity may depend on peak blood levels
Kanamycin	*Infants less than 2kg:* 15mg/kg/day IV/IM divided q12h for first week, then 20mg/kg/day divided q12h *Infants more than 2kg:* 20mg/kg/day IV/IM disease divided q12h for first week, then 30mg/kg/day divided q8h *Older children:* 15mg/kg/day IV/IM divided q12h	Ototoxic Potential for neuromuscular blockade following rapid infusion (administer slowly over 30 to 60min.) May aggravate pre-existing renal
Nitrofurantoin	5 to 7mg/kg/day po divided q6h Inappropriate for newborn	Nausea, vomiting Peripheral neuropathy Pulmonary infiltration with eosinophilia Haemolysis in G6PD deficiency
Penicillin G	25,000 to 50,000u/kg/day po divided q6h (1hr before or 2hrs after meals)	Hypersensitivity rashes Diarrhoea
Penicillin V phenoxymethyl-penicillin)	15 to 30mg/kg/day po divided q6h (1hr before or 2hrs after meals)	As for penicillin G
Sulphafurazole (sulfisoxazole)	120 to 150mg/kg/day po or IV divided q6h	Nausea, vomiting, rash Haemolysis in G6PD deficiency Kernicterus in newborn
Tobramycin	3 to 5mg/kg/day IV or IM divided q12h for newborns and q8h thereafter	As for gentamicin

Table III. Guide to the use of antibacterial drugs in the prophylaxis of paediatric urinary tract infections

Antibacterial drug	Dose and route	Side Effects
Co-trimoxazole (trimethoprim + sulpha- methoxazole in a 1:5 ratio)	10mg sulphamethoxazole/ kg/day po divided q12h	See table I
Hexamine (methenamine) mandelate or hippurate	50mg/kg/day po divided q8h	Nausea, vomiting, dysuria Breakthrough infection may occur (Vainrub and Musher, 1977)
Nitrofurantoin	2.5mg/kg administered as a single dose at bedtime Patients with urogenital abnormalities may require an extra dose (as above) in morning	See table I
Sulphafurazole (sulfisoxazole)	20 to 30mg/kg/day divided q8h	See table I

be repaired surgically, and children with frequent recurrences of infection, require chronic urinary antiseptic treatment. The objective of this type of therapy is to prevent serious ascending urinary tract infections with destruction of renal parenchyma and loss of kidney function. Patient compliance is critical and a variety of regimens are useful. These include co-trimoxazole, sulphonamides, nitrofurantoin and hexamine (methenamine) (see also section 2.6.2 and table III). For example, a single dose of nitrofurantoin at bedtime (2.5mg/kg) has been found to be effective in preventing recurrences in young girls with recurrent urinary tract infections but no underlying structural urinary tract abnormalities (Lohr et al., 1977). Caution is advised if hexamine is used (Vainrub and Musher, 1977). Breakthrough bacteriurias, symptomatic or not, should be treated aggressively for a two week period as discussed above.

3.6 Prognosis

The prognosis of pyelonephritis in childhood is improving, although much prospective study is still needed. The risk of acquiring renal damage and loss of function in infants and children with recurrent urinary tract infections without structural abnormalities should be minimal with careful attention to antiseptic therapy and detection of intercurrent infection. Patients with structural abnormalities and/or underlying neuromuscular or metabolic (i.e. nephrolithiasis) problems may have a poorer prognosis. Urine flow, repair of obstruction and avoidance of residual urine are essential.

In certain patients, progressive renal destruction due to repeated infection and poor functioning of surgical diversions or other host factors may lead to a chronic renal failure. The future prospects for these patients will depend on improved surgical and immunological approaches to renal and urinary tract transplantation surgery.

References

Bailey, R.R. and Abbott, G.D.: Treatment of urinary tract infection with a single dose of amoxycillin. Nephron 18: 316 (1977).

Bailey, R.R. and Abbott, G.D.: Treatment of urinary tract infection with a single dose of trimethoprim-sulfamethoxazole. Canadian Medical Association Journal 118: 551-552 (1978).

Barry, A.L.; Smith, P.B. and Turck, M.: Laboratory diagnosis of urinary tract infection. Cumitech 2, American Society of Microbiologists (1975).

Bowie, W.R.; Alexander, E.R.; Floyd, J.F.; Holmes, J.; Miller, Y. and Holmes, K.K.: Differential response of chlamydial and urea-plasma-associated urethritis to sulphafurazole (sulfisoxazole) and aminocyclitols. Lancet 2: 1276-1278 (1976).

Cohen, M.: Urinary tract infections in children. 1. Females aged 2 through 14, first two infections. Pediatrics 50: 271-278 (1972).

Dodge, W.F.; West, E.F. and Travis, L.B.: Bacteriuria in school children. American Journal of Diseases in Children 127: 364-370 (1974).

Du, J.N.H.: Colic as the sole symptom of urinary tract infection in infants. Canadian Medical Association Journal 115: 334-335 (1976).

Edelmann, C.M. Jr.; Ogwo, J.E.; Fine, B.P. and Martinez, A.B.: The prevalence of bacteriuria in full-term and premature newborn infants. Journal of Pediatrics 82: 125-132 (1973).

Fair, W.R. and Wehner, N.: Further observations on the antibacterial nature of prostatic fluid. Infection and Immunity 3: 494-495 (1971).

Forbes, P.A.; Drummond, K.N. and Nogrady, M.B.: Initial urinary tract infections. Journal of Pediatrics 75: 187-192 (1969).

Geist, R.W. and Antolak, S.J.: Interstitial cystitis in children. Journal of Urology 104: 922-925 (1969).

Gerstein, A.R.; Okun, R.; Gonick, H.C.; Wilner, H.I.; Kleeman, C.R. and Maxwell, M.H.: The prolonged use of methenamine hippurate in the treatment of chronic urinary tract infection. Journal of Urology 100: 767-771 (1968).

Gillenwater, J.Y.; Gleason, C.H.; Lohr, J.A. and Marion, D.: Home urine cultures by the dip-strip method: Results in 289 cultures. Pediatrics 58: 508-512 (1976).

Hallett, R.J.; Pead, L. and Maskell, R.: Urinary infection in boys. A three-year prospective study. Lancet 2: 1107-1110 (1976).

Harle, E.M.J.; Bullen, J.J. and Thomson, D.A.: Influence of estrogen on experimental pyelonephritis caused by Escherichia coli. Lancet 2: 283-286 (1975).

Holmes, K.K.; Handsfield, H.H.; Wang, S.P.; Wentworth, B.B.; Turck, M.; Anderson, J.B. and Alexander, E.R.: Etiology of nongonococcal urethritis. New England Journal of Medicine 292: 1199-1205 (1975).

Hulbert, J.: Gram-negative urinary infection treated with oral penicillin G. Lancet 2: 1216-1220 (1972).

Kaijser, B.: Immunology of Escherichia coli: K antigen and its relation to urinary-tract infection. Journal of Infectious Diseases 127: 670-677 (1973).

Kaijser, B.; Hanson, L.A.; Jodal, U.; Lidin-Janson, G. and Robbins, J.B.; Frequency of E. coli antigens in urinary-tract infections in children. Lancet 1: 663-666 (1977).

Karney, W.W.; Pedersen, A.H.B.; Nelson, M.; Adams, H.; Pfeifer, R.T. and Holmes, K.K.: Spectinomycin versus tetracycline for the treatment of gonorrhea. New England Journal of Medicine 296: 889-894 (1977).

Kellogg, D.S. Jr.; Holmes, K.K. and Hill, G.A.: Laboratory diagnosis of gonorrhea. Cumitech 4, American Society of Microbiologists (1976).

Klugo, R.C.; Anderson, J.A.; Reid, R.; Powell, I. and Cerny, J.C.: Xanthogranulomatous pyelonephritis in children. Journal of Urology 117: 350-352 (1977).

Kunin, C.M. Urinary tract infections in infancy. Journal of Pediatrics 86: 483-484 (1975).

Kunin, C.M.: Urinary tract infections in children. Hospital Practice 11: 91-98 (1976).

Lindberg, U.; Jodal, U.; Hanson, L.A. and Kaijser, B.: Asymptomatic bacteriuria in school girls. Acta Pediatrica Scandinavica 64: 574-580 (1975).

Lohr, J.A.; Nunley, D.H. Howards, S.S. and Ford, R.F.: Prevention of recurrent urinary tract infections in girls. Pediatrics 59: 562-565 (1977).

Marks, M.I.: Iatrogenic pneumaturia. Journal of Urology 106: 407-408 (1971).

Middleton, A.W., Jr. and Hendren, W.H.: Ileal conduits in children at the Massachusetts General Hospital from 1955 to 1970. Journal of Urology 115: 591-595 (1976).

Mou, T.W.: Effect of urine pH on the antibacterial activity of antibiotics and chemotherapeutic agents. Journal of Urology 87: 978-987 (1962).

Nelson, J.D.; Mohs, E.; Danjani, A.S. and Plotkin, S.A.: Gonorrhea in preschool- and school-aged children. Journal of the American Medical Association 236: 1359-1364 (1976).

Numazaki, Y.; Kumasaka, T.; Yano, N.; Yamanaka, M.; Miyazawa, T.; Takai, S. and Ishida, N.: Further study on acute hemorrhagic cystitis due to adenovirus type II. New England Journal of Medicine 289: 344-347 (1973).

Orikasa, S.; Koyanagi, T.; Motomura, M.; Kudo, T.; Togashi, M. and Tsuji, I.: Experience with non-sterile, intermittent self-catheterization. Journal of Urology 115: 141-142 (1976).

Pryles, C.V. and Lustik, B.: Laboratory diagnosis of urinary tract infection. Paediatric Clinics of North America 18: 233-244 (1971).

Savage, D.C.L.; Adler, K.; Howie, G. and Wilson, M.I.: Controlled trial of therapy in covert bacteriuria of childhood. Lancet 1: 358-361 (1975).

Saxena, S.R.; Laurance, B.M. and Shaw, D.G.: The justification for early radiological investigations of urinary-tract infection in children. Lancet 2: 403-404 (1975).

Shopfner, C.E.: Modern concepts of lower urinary tract obstruction in pediatric patients. Pediatrics 45: 194-196 (1970).

Shore, W.B. and Winkelstein, J.A.: Nonvenereal transmission of gonococcal infections to children. Journal of Pediatrics 79: 661-663 (1971).

Welch, T.R.; Forbes, P.A.; Drummond, K.N. and Nogrady, M.B.: Recurrent urinary tract infection in girls. Archives of Diseases of Childhood 51: 114-119 (1976).

Wilkinson, A.E.; Seth, A.D. and Rodin, P.: Infection with penicillinase-producing gonococcus. British Medical Journal 2: 1233-1235 (1976).

Chapter V

Skin and Wound Infections

M.I. Marks

The most common aetiological agents involved in skin and wound infections in infants and children are *Staphylococcus aureus* and *Streptococcus pyogenes*. These frequently manifest as impetigo, furunculosis, cellulitis and wound infections. Other important bacterial pathogens include *Haemophilus influenzae* which causes cellulitis, and Gram-negative bacteria such as *E. coli* and *Pseudomonas aeruginosa* which are responsible for wound infections.

Host characteristics determine the type of superficial infections encountered. For example, leukaemic patients may have Pseudomonas infections of the skin (echthyma gangrenosum). Patients with indwelling chest tubes may have wound infections due to *Staphylococcus epidermidis,* and burn patients may develop superficial infections with a variety of bacteria.

This chapter will deal with selected common bacterial skin and wound infections. Less common bacterial and mycobacterial infections such as leprosy and tuberculosis and infections due to atypical mycobacteria will not be discussed.

1. Impetigo

The most common manifestations of group A streptococcal infections of the skin in children are lesions clinically characterised as impetigo.

1.1 Pathogenesis

The pathogenesis of impetigo is interesting in that group A *Streptococcus pyogenes* often colonises normal skin before any lesions are seen. Subsequent development of skin lesions and colonisation of the respiratory tract have been documented (Dudding et al., 1970). *Staphylococcus aureus* is commonly found in impetiginous lesions in association with *Streptococcus pyogenes*, but is usually (though not always) thought to be a secondary invader. Therapeutic trials have indicated that the *Staphylococcus aureus*, although frequently resistant to penicillin, disappears along with the *Streptococcus pyogenes* when penicillin therapy is given (Wannamaker, 1970). However, staphylococci may be the primary invaders in some instances (and indeed, in some parts of the world, the pathogenic role of these two organisms appears to be reversed with staphylococcal impetigo being the most commonly encountered) and the distinctive bullous form of impetigo (see section 1.4) is of staphylococcal origin.

1.2 Clinical Features and Diagnosis

The clinical diagnosis is made on the basis of lesions which are heaped up and rapidly progressive from a red papular appearance to a weeping lesion with a serous exudate. These may be localised to a specific area of the body or generalised. The degree of involvement of the skin, as well as adjacent lymphadenitis determines the degree of systemic toxicity. The laboratory diagnosis consists of culturing group A *Streptococcus pyogenes* from a scraping taken from the base of a lesion or from material obtained by unroofing an early papular lesion. *Staphylococcus aureus* is also often grown from a culture taken from the superficial area of this lesion.

Sequelae of this infection include the development of glomerulonephritis subsequent to infections of the skin with nephritogenic strains of streptococci (Ferrieri et al., 1970). This results from the renal glomerular deposition of immune complexes containing streptococcal antigen, streptococcal antibody and complement.

1.3 Treatment

The therapy of impetigo is controversial when there are only a few lesions present. The evidence accumulated, however, suggests that systemic penicillin therapy in combination with improved personal hygiene is associated with the most rapid resolution of disease and sterilisation of the lesions (Ruby and Nelson, 1973). The possibility that glomerulonephritis may be prevented by the use of penicillin therapy is an added, but unproven, incentive (Ferrieri et al., 1970). There is evidence that the use of hexachlorophane and/or topical antibiotic therapy is not as efficacious as systemic penicillin therapy; nor is it necessary to add these therapies to penicillin (Ruby and Nelson, 1973). Penicillin, soap bathing, improvement in general hygiene and cleaning and trimming of finger-nails are sufficient.

The presence of adjacent lymphadenitis and systemic toxicity makes it mandatory to treat with penicillin. A lack of response to penicillin therapy in the severely infected patient should stimulate a search for a secondary infection, such as staphylococcal lymphadenitis. Other close contacts with similar lesions should also be diagnosed and treated as the cycle of repetitive streptococcal skin infections may not be interrupted by the treatment of only one family member. Impetigo in a household is often an indicator of sub-standard hygiene and may be an important clue regarding other preventable health problems.

1.4 Bullous Impetigo

When the lesions of impetigo take on a bullous appearance, *Staphylococcus aureus* is the most common cause. The diagnosis may be confirmed by Gram stain of the fluid within the bullous lesion which demonstrates polymorphonuclear leucocytes and Gram-positive cocci. Occasionally, these lesions do not contain staphylococci and the site of colonisation may be at a distance (for example, the anterior nares). The clinical picture should alert the clinician to the staphylococcal aetiology and treatment in this situation should be with an antistaphylococcal drug. We prefer to use cloxacillin 100mg/kg/day or dicloxacillin 50mg/kg/day orally (divided 6-hourly). If untreated, the lesions may possibly extend to other areas of the skin and even to a clinical picture of staphylococcal scalded skin syndrome (Lillibridge et al., 1972).

2. Staphylococcal Scalded Skin Syndrome

This syndrome is also known as toxic epidermal necrolysis, Lyell's disease or Ritter's disease of the newborn.

2.1 Pathogenesis

The condition is due to an exotoxin derived from *Staphylococcus aureus* (usually phage group II) [Elias et al., 1975; Lillibridge et al., 1972]. The toxin has been called exfoliatoxin as its major manifestation is exfoliation of the skin due to intercellular cleavage and cell separation in the epidermis (Lillibridge et al., 1972).

2.2 Clinical Features and Diagnosis

Manifestations in children include a scarlatinaform rash, bullous impetigo (see also section 1.4) and generalised exfoliation (Lillibridge et al., 1972). More commonly in adults, and occasionally in children, allergies to drugs and other agents may be responsible for the latter syndrome. Nevertheless, staphylococci account for most of the disease seen in children and the newborn.

The diagnosis is confirmed by culture of *Staphylococcus aureus* from the anterior nares, and occasionally from the skin sites of infections. The most important evidence would be the lack of a recognisable allergen in the history and a favourable response to antistaphylococcal penicillin therapy.

2.3 Treatment

When encountered clinically, antistaphylococcal therapy (e.g. cloxacillin) should be started immediately. The intravenous route is recommended for the scalded skin syndrome although oral therapy may be used in localised lesions such as bullous impetigo. Nursing care is an important component of therapy as the skin may easily cleave off apparently normal areas simply due to pressure (Nikolsky's sign). Therefore, avoidance of binding and any pressure on the rest of the skin surface is important.

The patient does not usually require other topical therapy and secondary bacterial infections and extreme fluid losses, as are encountered with burns, do not complicate therapy. Corticosteroids are not indicated in the staphylococcal scalded skin syndrome.

3. Cellulitis

3.1 Pathogenesis

Bacterial causes of cellulitis include *Streptococcus pyogenes* group A, *Staphylococcus aureus* and *Haemophilus influenzae*. Occasionally, *Streptococcus pneumoniae* may cause similar lesions, particularly in the area of the face and eye. Under the age of four years *Haemophilus influenzae* is as frequent a cause of cellulitis as is *Streptococcus pyogenes* group A (Haynes and Cramblett, 1967). The pathogenesis of many of these lesions is unclear, but is often related to a small and superficial abrasion and/or respiratory focus. The latter is particularly relevant to those infections seen about the eye and those over the sinuses (Haynes and Cramblett, 1967).

3.2 Clinical Features and Diagnosis

The diagnosis of cellulitis in infants and children depends upon the clinical appearance of a tender, oedematous, erythematous and warm lesion on the skin. If this is over a joint or on an extremity, there may be decreased mobility. Occasionally cellulitis may have a sharply demarcated border with a raised margin characteristic of *Streptococcus pyogenes* group A and at other times may have a bluish discoloration said to be characteristic of *Haemophilus influenzae*. These descriptions, however, should not be relied upon as a guide to therapy.

The diagnosis is confirmed in the laboratory by Gram stain of a small amount of fluid obtained by intradermal inoculation of the advancing border of the cellulitis and culture of the same fluid. A superficial skin swab, after preparation of the skin, but before obtaining the above culture, is often useful in helping the clinician to differentiate superficial skin colonisation due to *Staphylococcus epidermidis* and/or *Staphylococcus aureus* from the infecting pathogens. This procedure should be followed by a blood culture and therapy subsequently initiated; cultures of the nasopharynx and throat are not useful in this situation. 'Streptozyme' or other tests of antistreptococcal antibody may be used to diagnose streptococcal skin infections in retrospect. Negative findings, however, do not eliminate the possibility of streptococcal infections.

Orbital cellulitis is a specific expression of cellulitis and requires extra care in diagnosis and therapy. Additional diagnostic measures should include Gram stain and culture of the exudate from the infected eye and similar examination of any purulent drainage from the ipsilateral naris.

3.3 Treatment

Parenteral antibiotics are almost always indicated in orbital cellulitis and therapy effective against *Haemophilus influenzae* should be added in patients under the age of 4 years. Intravenous cloxacillin in a dosage of 200mg/kg/day (divided 6-hourly) plus ampicillin 200mg/kg/day (divided 6-hourly) is a combination which will effectively treat most staphylococcal, streptococcal and Haemophilus infections causing cellulitis of the orbit and other facial areas. Chloramphenicol 75mg/kg/day (divided 6-hourly) may be required if the infection is caused by ampicillin resistant strains of *Haemophilus influenzae*.

Cellulitis often occurs secondary to abrasions. When these are well localised and systemic toxicity is minimal, it is justifiable to initiate therapy with oral penicillin V. Gram stain, culture results and clinical response will determine future therapy in this type of patient. Resolution of toxicity should ensue within 48 hours. Occasionally, oedema of the extremity is seen with streptococcal disease due to involvement of the lymphatics. Oedema, in the absence of progression of the other signs of inflammation, locally and systemically, should not suggest a different pathogenesis or aetiology. When the patient is more toxic it is safer to administer antistaphylococcal and antistreptococcal therapy by the intravenous route. We use cloxacillin 200mg/kg/day. *H. influenzae* should also be considered in the aetiology of cellulitis in children under 4 years of age, and ampicillin or amoxycillin given.

Careful examination should be carried out in all patients with cellulitis for lymphadenitis, lymphangiitis and systemic manifestations of these localised infections. Additionally, patients with orbital cellulitis should have a careful examination of the eye and retrobulbar area to eliminate the possibility of abscess formation, infectious neuritis and thrombosis. Follow-up should include visual acuity and examination of the sinuses for blockage by polyps and other predisposing factors. Lack of resolution of a cellulitis overlying a sinus should alert the clinician to examine the sinus and teeth radiographically and clinically for evidence of abscess formation, osteomyelitis, etc. This is also true of cellulitis over-lying bone and joints. Any clinical and laboratory signs suggestive of septicaemia and/or meningitis should be pursued aggressively to avoid misdiagnosis of cellulitis as being an indication of only a superficial infection.

4. Furunculosis

Furunculosis is a common feature of acne vulgaris in teenagers, which will be discussed below (section 5).

4.1 Pathogenesis

Occasionally, hair follicles or other skin appendages become infected, most commonly by *Staphylococcus aureus*, with the appearance of specific abscess-type lesions such as paronychia, boils and furuncules. The pathogenesis of these lesions is sometimes unclear and they may reappear in crop-like fashion — the so-called 'idiopathic recurrent furunculosis syndrome'. Regardless of clinical expression, the diagnosis and therapy are often similar. Most patients who have difficulty with furunculosis carry *Staphylococcus aureus* in their anterior nares of the same phage group as is present in the infected lesion. This may be a short term carriage and may cause only a single infection, or it may be present in this site for a longer period of time and be associated with recurrent lesions in the same place or at different locations. Occasionally, the site of carriage is in the anus or axilla. Gram stain of lesion fluid reveals bacteria in association with polymorphonuclear leucocytes. These are easily cultured on routine media.

4.2 Treatment

Staphylococcus aureus should always be considered resistant to penicillin in the initial therapy of serious infections. Therapy can be subsequently adjusted to penicillin alone if the infecting organism is demonstrated to be penicillin sensitive by appropriate laboratory tests. Drainage is a most important first-line of therapy for localised staphylococcal abscesses. Antibiotics such as cloxacillin 100mg/kg/day or dicloxacillin 50mg/kg/day (divided 6-hourly), may be administered orally to supplement drainage procedures in most localised lesions.

Furunculosis may lead to invasive staphylococcal disease in some patients. Systemic signs and symptoms should alert the clinician to the possibility.

4.2.1 Treatment of Recurrent Lesions

Occasionally, patients have recurrent lesions in a specific site or in a generalised fashion. These patients may benefit from a programme of diagnosis and therapy as follows:

1) *Definition of the carriage site.* This is an important part of the programme. Cultures should be obtained from the infected lesion and from other sites in the body such as the anterior nares, normal skin, axillae and anal region. These cultures should be repeated when the patient is well and free from infection. All staphylococcal isolates should be phage grouped; the finding of the identical phage group in a typical carrier site is very useful to the clinician (Strauss et al., 1969).

2) *Specific therapy.* The clinician should try to define a symptomatic prodrome for the infections, whereupon he can institute topical antibiotic therapy (e.g. bacitracin ointment) to the site of carriage, together with hexachlorophane baths and systemic antistaphylococcal therapy.

3) *Further investigations.* Investigation of patients for immunological deficiencies including abnormal phagocyte functions, morphology and numbers, agamaglobulinaemia, diabetes mellitus, hypocomplementaemia and other host defects are warranted, but often not fruitful.

Investigational techniques for eradication of the staphylococcus from such hosts by colonisation with 'non-pathogenic' strains of *Staphylococcus aureus*, use of autogenous vaccines (Smith, 1970), gammaglobulin injections etc., are usually not necessary. These procedures may have adverse reactions (Houck et al., 1972) and cannot be recommended on the basis of investigations available at the present time.

Patients with recurrent staphylococcal furunculosis and their families require reassurance and explanation about the self-limiting nature of the condition and the probability that children will outgrow the problem over several months of observation and careful therapy.

5. Acne Vulgaris

5.1 Pathogenesis

Acne vulgaris is an inflammatory condition of the sebaceous glands common in adolescents and in patients receiving adrenal corticosteroid therapy. Bacteria isolated

Table I. Summary of the treatment of common skin and wound infections in infants and children

---

1. *Impetigo*
    a) Systemic penicillin therapy plus improved personal hygiene adequate
    b) Topical antibiotics not required
    c) Treat close contacts with similar lesions
    d) *Bullous impetigo* (most commonly due to *S. aureus*): use an antistaphylococcal penicillin (e.g. cloxacillin, 100mg/kg/day or dicloxacillin, 50mg/kg/day orally)
2. *Staphylococcal scalded skin syndrome* (toxic epidermal necrolysis, Lyell's disease, Ritter's disease of the newborn)
    a) Start IV antistaphylococcal penicillin (e.g. cloxacillin) immediately
    b) Nursing care important; avoid binding and pressure on the rest of the skin surface
    c) Topical therapy not required
3. *Cellulitis*
    a) *Orbital cellulitis:* Give IV cloxacillin (200mg/kg/day) plus ampicillin (200mg/kg/day)
    b) Cellulitis with minimal systemic toxicity: initiate therapy with penicillin V; further therapy is guided by Gram stain, culture results and clinical response. Use ampicillin or amoxycillin in children < 4 years of age
    c) When patient is more toxic, give IV cloxacillin (200mg/kg/day). Add ampicillin in children < 4 years of age
    d) Careful follow-up necessary in all patients to detect abscess formation, osteomyelitis, etc.
4. *Furunculosis*
    a) Use antistaphylococcal penicillin initially (e.g. cloxacillin, 100mg/kg/day or dicloxacillin, 50mg/kg/day orally)
    b) Change to penicillin if infecting organism subsequently shown to be penicillin sensitive
    c) Drainage important for localised abscesses
    d) *Recurrent lesions:* Define carriage site and institute topical therapy (e.g. bacitracin ointment); investigate patient for immunological deficiency and other host defects. Give antistaphylococcal penicillin at first sign of new lesions and continue until 48 hrs after resolution
5. *Acne vulgaris*
    a) Long term tetracycline therapy (250mg/day) indicated in moderate to severe cases and those not responding adequately to topical measures (e.g. benzoyl peroxide or retinoic acid)
    b) Erythromycin is an effective alternative to tetracycline
6. *Wound infections*
    a) Treat as for staphylococcal infections and cellulitis. Clinical course and results of aerobic and anaerobic cultures may guide further therapy
    b) Antibiotic prophylaxis useful for many surgical procedures (e.g. gastrointestinal resection and abscess drainage)

---

from these lesions include the diphtheroid *Propionibacterium acnes* and *Staphylococcus epidermidis* (Marples and Izumi, 1970; Leyden and Kligman, 1976). The most important aspects of pathogenesis are determined by the host and include androgenic stimulation of sebaceous gland activity and irritation by fatty acids produced by the action of bacterial lipases.

5.2 Treatment

Tetracycline 250mg/day is effective in reducing inflammation by inhibiting these bacterial lipases. Tetracycline therapy is recommended in moderate to severe cases and in patients not responding adequately to therapy with simple hygienic procedures and comedone extraction (Reisner, 1973) or to treatment with topical benzoyl peroxide or retinoic acid (tretinoin) preparations. Low dosages (effective because of high concentration of drug in sebaceous glands) should be used to avoid drug toxicity. Erythromycin may be used as an alternative to tetracycline.

Gram-negative folliculitis is an uncommon but serious complication of acne vulgaris heralded by the appearance of increasing pustule formation and confirmed by the culture of Gram-negative bacteria from the lesions (Leyden et al., 1973). Tetracycline therapy should be interrupted and specific antibiotic and drainage therapies instituted. Antibiotic therapy is guided by culture and sensitivity testing.

Complications of long term low dose tetracycline therapy include Candida vaginitis (especially in girls also taking oral contraceptives) and skin photosensitivity reactions.

6. Wound Infections

Approximately 5% of infants and children subjected to 'clean' surgical procedures have staphylococcal and/or Gram-negative wound infections.

6.1 Diagnosis and Treatment

Diagnosis and treatment of these infections should follow the same guidelines as outlined for staphylococcal skin infections and cellulitis. Most antibiotics including penicillin and ampicillin diffuse well into wounds (Alexander et al., 1973). Infections resulting from contaminated lesions such as a ruptured appendix may be more complicated. These infections are often more resistant to therapy with conventional antistaphylococcal and antistreptococcal drugs and may require drainage and antibiotics effective against anaerobic bacteria (e.g. chloramphenicol 75mg/kg/day divided 6-hourly orally or IV, or metronidazole 20 to 30mg/kg/day divided 8-hourly). Cultures from suspected lesions should include anaerobic examination; however, anaerobes as a sole infecting bacteria are rare.

6.2 Antibiotic Prophylaxis

Antibiotic and/or antiseptic prophylaxis are useful for many surgical procedures, including gastrointestinal resection and abscess drainage (Gilmore et al.,

1973; Editorial, 1976; Chodak and Plaut, 1978). Preliminary evidence suggests that metronidazole may be useful in decreasing the incidence of anaerobic wound infections following anorectal and colorectal surgery (Brass et al., 1978), although further controlled studies are needed to evaluate this drug in appendicitis and other surgical conditions in children. These measures, however, must not be used as a substitute for careful aseptic and surgical techniques. Antibiotics should be administered immediately after appropriate cultures are taken at the time of operation and should be continued for 48 hours after surgery. This short term usage of antibiotics is associated with the least risk of bacterial superinfection.

Direct installation of antibiotics or antiseptics (such as povidone iodine) into the wound in the form of powders or sprays has also been associated with a decrease in wound infections (Editorial, 1976). The use of such programmes needs to be combined with careful surveillance for emergence of resistant organisms and documentation of improvement in wound infection rates.

7. Special Hosts: Treatment Considerations

The most common pathogens of infancy and childhood responsible for skin and wound infections have been discussed above. Specific hosts however, may require special consideration.

7.1 Neonates

In the newborn, the peculiar susceptibility of the host and exposure to maternal and nursery bacterial flora create a complicated situation. Skin and wound infections in this age group require precise laboratory identification including Gram smears and careful culture and susceptibility testing. Prophylactic techniques including hexachlorophane washing have been associated with a decrease in infection rates, but unacceptable toxicity in certain situations (Gowdy and Ulsamer, 1976; Kensit, 1975). The use of hexachlorophane, in the face of its toxicity, for newborn nurseries, especially in premature infants, warrants careful control. The application of triple-dye to the umbilicus of newborns and the use of gentle soap and water, or a single hexachlorophane bath with adequate rinsing, is usually adequate. More frequent hexachlorophane bathing is best reserved for control of nursery staphylococcal outbreaks.

7.2 Eczema and Burn Patients

Other examples of abnormal hosts include patients with eczema and burns. The former have difficulty with staphylococcal and streptococcal infections which may be related to underlying abnormality of the skin, although recent evidence indicates these patients may have abnormal phagocytes as well (Khan, 1975). The burn patient is most susceptible to *Streptococcus pyogenes* group A infections in the first week after burn and to Gram-negative infections thereafter. The use of penicillin prophylaxis in the first few days and topical antiseptic treatment thereafter is reasonable. Povidone iodine, silver sulphadiazine, silver nitrate and mafenide have all been associated with a decrease in the quantity and severity of burn wound infections (Moncrief, 1973). These techniques are not without complications however, and need frequent monitoring (Lowbury et al., 1976; Pietsch and Meakins, 1976). They should be used as an adjunct to the general care of the patients. Recent evidence indicates that optimal nutrition, careful debridement and rapid grafting of these wounds are even more important than antiseptic methods for prevention of infection and fatality due to sepsis. Parenteral antibiotic therapy should be guided by clinical signs of infection supported by quantitative bacterial cultures. These latter are most predictive of infection when they are obtained by the skin biopsy technique and quantitated.

Skin and wound infections in these patients illustrate how knowledge of some of the characteristics of the host are critical in evaluating the potential manifestations of invading bacteria.

References

Alexander, J.W.; Sykes, N.S.; Mitchell, M.M. and Fisher, M.W.: Concentration of selected intravenously administered antibiotics in experimental surgical wounds. Journal of Trauma 13: 423 (1973).

Brass, C.; Richards, G.K.; Ruedy, J.; Prentis, J. and Hinchley, E.J.: The effect of metronidazole on the incidence of postoperative wound infection in elective colon surgery. American Journal of Surgery 135: 91-95 (1978).

Chodak, G.W. and Plaut, M.E.: Use of systemic antibiotics for prophylaxis in surgery. A critical review. Archives of Surgery 112: 326-334 (1977).

Dudding, B.A.; Burnett, J.W.; Chapman, S.S. and Wannamaker, L.W.: The role of normal skin in the spread of streptococcal pyoderma. Journal of Hygiene (Cambridge) 68: 19 (1970).

Editorial: Prophylactic povidone iodine. Lancet 1: 73 (1976).

Elias, P.M.; Fritsch, P.; Dahl, M.V. and Wolff, K.: Staphylococcal toxic epidermal necrolysis: Pathogenesis and studies on the subcellular site of action of exfoliatin. Journal of Investigative Dermatology 65: 501 (1975).

Ferrieri, P.; Dajani, A.S.; Chapman, S.S.; Jensen, J.B. and Wannamaker, L.W.: Appearance of nephritis associated with type 57 streptococcal impetigo in North America. New England Journal of Medicine 283: 832 (1970).

Gilmore, O.J.A.; Martin, T.D.M. and Fletcher, B.N.: Prevention of wound infection after appendicectomy. Lancet 2: 220 (1973).

Gowdy, J.M. and Ulsamer, A.G.: Hexachlorophene lesions in newborn infants. American Journal of Diseases in Children 130: 247 (1976).

Haynes, R.W. and Cramblett, H.G.: Acute Ethmoiditis. Its relationship to orbital cellulitis. American Journal of Diseases in Children 114: 261 (1967).

Houck, P.W.; Nelson, J.D. and Kay, J.L.: Fatal septicemia due to *Staphylococcus aureus* 502A. American Journal of Diseases in Children 123: 45 (1972).

Kahn, G.: Symposium on pediatric allergy. Eczematoid eruptions in children. Pediatric Clinics of North America 22: 203 (1975).

Kensit, J.G.: Hexachlorophane: Toxicity and effectiveness in prevention of sepsis in neonatal units. Journal of Antimicrobial Chemotherapy 1: 263 (1975).

Leyden, J.J. and Kligman, A.M.: Acne vulgaris: New concepts in pathogenesis and treatment. Drugs 12: 292-300 (1976).

Leyden, J.J.; Marples, R.R.; Mills, O.H. and Kligman, A.M.: Gram-negative folliculitis — a complication of antibiotic therapy in acne vulgaris. British Journal of Dermatology 88: 533 (1973).

Lillibridge, C.B.; Melish, M.E. and Glasgow, L.A.: Site of action of exfoliative toxin in the staphylococcal scalded-skin syndrome. Pediatrics 50: 728 (1972).

Lowbury, E.J.L.; Babb, J.R.; Bridges, K. and Jackson, D.M.: Topical chemoprophylaxis with silver sulphadiazine and silver nitrate chlorhexidine creams: Emergence of sulphonamide-resistant Gram-negative bacilli. British Medical Journal 1: 493 (1976).

Marples, R.R. and Izumi, A.K.: Bacteriology of pustular acne. Journal of Investigative Dermatology 54: 252 (1970).

Moncrief, J.A.: Burns. New England Journal of Medicine 288: 444 (1973).

Pietsch, J. and Meakins, J.L.: Complications of povidone-iodine absorption in topically treated burn patients. Lancet 1: 280 (1976).

Reisner, R.M.: Acne vulgaris. Pediatric Clinics of North America 20: 851 (1973).

Ruby, R.J. and Nelson, J.D.: The influence of hexachlorophene scrubs on the response to placebo or penicillin therapy in impetigo. Pediatrics 52: 854 (1973).

Smith, D.T.: Autogenous vaccines in theory and in practice. Archives of Internal Medicine 125: 344 (1970).

Strauss, W.G.; Maibach, H.I. and Shinefield, H.R.: Bacterial interference treatment of recurrent furunculosis. 2. Demonstration of the relationship of strain to pathogenicity. Journal of the American Medical Association 208: 861 (1969).

Wannamaker, L.W.: Differences between streptococcal infections of the throat and of the skin. New England Journal of Medicine 282: 23 (1970).

Chapter VI

Infections of the Skeletal System

G.A. Ahronheim

Suppurative infections of the developing skeletal system, through their effects on growth, symmetry, posture and gait, may result in permanent disfigurement or crippling of an otherwise healthy child, especially when tardily or inadequately treated. Because of their frequency in childhood and their potential sequelae, a haematogenous osteomyelitis and septic arthritis will be emphasised in this chapter.

1. Osteomyelitis

Acute haematogenous osteomyelitis is predominantly a disease of the growing child, although a distinct clinical pattern has evolved among intravenous drug abusers.

1.1 Pathogenesis and Aetiology

Pyogenic bacteria gain access to the blood stream at remote sites, most commonly from cutaneous infections but also from respiratory and gastrointestinal loci; if inadequately cleared by natural host defences such as the reticuloendothelial system of the lung and spleen, they may become entrapped in the anatomically and physiologically unique subepiphyseal vasculature of growing bones (Waldvogel et al., 1970). Antecedent mild trauma to the overlying area is a frequent part of the clinical history; its role, if any, in the pathogenesis of the infection remains to be defined. Bacterial multiplication and the evoked inflammatory responses spread via the osseous and medullary channels. Bone necrosis and demineralisation ensue, and suppuration may eventually rupture through the cortex and elevate the periosteum, with further spread and vascular compromise.

In the neonate, metaphyseal infection can traverse the growth plate via vascular channels and involve the epiphysis. The epiphysis and the joint space are also at risk of infection via the transcortical or subperiosteal routes; in either instance, blood supply to the epiphysis may be compromised and the epiphysis is subject to the dual risk of ischaemia and/or infection (Ogden and Lister, 1975). Reparative processes include the laying down of new bone and sequestration of avascular dead bone, but are not always completely successful as the existence of chronic osteomyelitis testifies.

Acute haematogenous osteomyelitis in children is usually caused by coagulase-positive staphylococci (*S. aureus*) which in most series accounts for well over half the cases, and at least 75 % of cases in which a bacteriological diagnosis is achieved. Haemolytic streptococci, principally group A *Strep. pyogenes*, account for another 5 to 10 % of cases. *Haemophilus influenzae* is responsible for another few percent in the age group below approximately 5 years, but is not as common as might be expected from its high frequency in other bacteraemic diseases of childhood (Epidemiological Research Laboratory, 1976). Pneumococcal osteomyelitis is now rare, encountered principally in persons with sickle cell anaemia.

Gram-negative enteric bacilli are becoming recognised more frequently, especially in sickle cell disease [in which salmonellae and other enteric bacilli are recognised to be particularly common (Barrett-Connor, 1971; Engh et al., 1974)], in metastatic bone seeding from bacteraemic salmonellosis, secondary osteomyelitis (Fitzgerald., 1975), and puncture wounds of the foot (not haematogenous disease *sensu strictu*) where *Pseudomonas aeruginosa* must be suspected in the presence of osteomyelitis (Brand and Black, 1974; Miller and Semian, 1975; Minnefor et al., 1971). Neonatal osteomyelitis, reviewed in chapter VIII, might have been expected to commonly involve Gram-negative organisms because of their frequent implication in neonatal sepsis; however, most reviews indicate that *S. aureus* predominates over other organisms such as coliforms, *Pseudomonas*, streptococci and gonococci (Weissberg et al., 1974). Not to be overlooked in the differential diagnosis of neonatal osteomyelitis is the periostitis caused by congenital infections such as syphilis.

Subacute and chronic osteomyelitis are frequently staphylococcal but may be culture-negative (Gledhill, 1973; Season and Miller, 1976; Waldvogel et al., 1970). Careful bacteriological study, perhaps including the use of hypertonic media to recover cell wall defective bacteria, should nevertheless not be omitted.

1.2 Clinical Features

Most common in children less than 10 years of age, and at least twice as frequent in boys as in girls, haematogenous osteomyelitis occurs in the distal femur, proximal tibia, and proximal humerus in about 75 % of cases; other long bones may also be affected, the flat and round bones being involved relatively infrequently. Although variable in presentation, the most common manifestations of osteomyelitis include local pain, tenderness, favouring of the involved part and fever. In the younger child and infant, unwillingness to use an extremity may be the crucial clue to explain undiagnosed fever, irritability, poor feeding and lethargy.

Except for point tenderness, physical signs of inflammation — local swelling, erythema, etc. — may take several days to appear. Peripheral leucocytosis and an elevated erythrocyte sedimentation rate are helpful but non-specific haematological findings.

1.3 Diagnosis

Although radiographic evidence of bone rarefaction and periosteal reaction is ordinarily not seen before the second week of illness, a careful examination of x-rays early in the course may reveal highly suggestive soft tissue changes as early as the third day (Capitanio and Kirkpatrick, 1970). Xeroradiography has been reported as demonstrating these early changes even more clearly (Crane et al., 1975). Recent work indicates that radioisotope scans may be a very valuable tool in the early diagnosis of osteomyelitis. Technetium labelled 'bone-seeking' radiopharmaceuticals such as ^{99m}Tc-diphosphonate appear to concentrate in areas of bone where local blood flow, metabolism and osteoblastic activity are increased; asymmetric bone uptake of these tracers may be the earliest confirmatory evidence of osteomyelitis, perhaps as early as the first 24 hours of illness (Handmaker and Leonards, 1976; Letts et al., 1975; Paul and Gilday, 1975; Treves et al., 1976). Not infrequently, soft tissue inflammation may overlie the suspect bone, complicating evaluation; the use of combined blood pool and bone scans with technetium has been suggested to differentiate between cellulitis and underlying osteomyelitis (Gilday and Paul, 1974).

Another problem which must be distinguished from osteomyelitis is bone infarction due to sickle cell anaemia, a disorder in which both occur with disturbing frequency (Diggs, 1967; Engh et al., 1974; Karayalcin et al., 1975). The early scintigraphic picture of bone infarction may be distinct, and immediate scans have been recommended to permit differentiation of infarction from infection (Lutzker et al., 1976).

The importance of accurate bacteriological diagnosis cannot be over-emphasised. Successful management may depend on optimal choice of antibiotics, based on detailed susceptibility testing of the patient's organism. We recommend multiple blood cultures, with early attempted needle aspiration of the subperiosteal space or a radiographically manifest bone lesion; blood culture should be repeated after manipulation or instrumentation. Gram stain of the aspirated material should reveal polymorphonuclear leucocytes, and organisms may be recognised on smear; the material should be quickly and carefully inoculated into appropriate culture media. If direct aspiration is unproductive, local lavage of the suspicious area with a small quantity of sterile non-bacteriostatic saline may yield diagnostic material. Bedside investigation includes a search for and appropriate attention to associated infection elsewhere — e.g. an obvious pyoderma. Under ideal circumstances, preliminary isolation and partial identification may be available from these cultures in less than 24 hours.

1.4 Treatment

1.4.1 Initial Therapy

Without specific aetiological clues, the predominance of staphylococci in osteomyelitis makes the inclusion of a penicillinase resistant β-lactam drug (e.g. an antistaphylococcal penicillin or a cephalosporin) mandatory in initial therapy. We use cloxacillin 150 to 200mg/kg/day in 4 to 6 divided doses intravenously. The IV route is strongly recommended during the first days and weeks of treatment to ensure reliable serum levels of the drug. The majority of streptococci are sensitive to levels achievable with these doses; therapy can be changed to the most appropriate drug — e.g. penicillin G for *Strep. pyogenes* — when bacteriological identification is complete.

In appropriate clinical circumstances as discussed above, or when Gram-negative rods are seen on Gram stain, ampicillin (150 to 200mg/kg/day in 4 to 6 divided doses IV) is used initially, in conjunction with an aminoglycoside (e.g. kanamycin 20mg/kg/day or gentamicin 5 to 7mg/kg/day in 2 divided doses IM or IV). Gentamicin should be used if *Pseudomonas* is suspected; kanamycin is equally effective if a non-nosocomial coliform is likely. The increasing recognition of Gram-negative pathogens resistant to both these drugs however, stresses the importance of *in vitro* susceptibility testing and a probable eventual role for newer aminoglycosides such as amikacin, tobramycin or sisomicin. (Because of potential ototoxicity and nephrotoxicity, baseline audiometry and renal studies should be obtained as early as practicable if aminoglycosides are used.) Therapy of Pseudomonas infection may require a combination of gentamicin and carbenicillin (300 to 400mg/kg/day in 6 divided doses IV) to take advantage of possible antibiotic synergism which may be demonstrated *in vitro* and, as in a recent study with sisomicin, *in vivo* (van Wingerden et al., 1974). Carbenicillin should not be used alone because of the likelihood of emergence of resistance *in vivo*, a phenomenon which combination therapy appears to prevent.

1.4.2 Alternative Therapy

Documented penicillin hypersensitivity necessitates alternative therapy. Cephalosporins are frequently a good substitute for penicillins, but caution is required in their use since cross sensitivity may be found in up to 10% of penicillin-allergic patients, and because published experience with cephalosporins in childhood osteomyelitis is limited (Pickering et al., 1974). Macrolide antibiotics have been used with some success: a recent study of clindamycin in children with osteomyelitis and septic arthritis due to Gram-positive organisms (Feigin et al., 1975) found good early results with relatively brief IV therapy followed by several weeks of oral therapy. However, the possibility of serious gastrointestinal side effects limits the use of clindamycin (Tedesco et al., 1974).

The successful use of fusidic acid in skeletal infections has also been reported (Blockley and McAllister, 1972; McAllister, 1974).

1.4.3 Duration of Therapy

The optimum duration of antibiotic therapy of osteomyelitis remains an unsettled issue. Some authors have achieved what they consider to be satisfactory results with only brief (up to 7 to 14 days) IV therapy followed by several weeks of oral therapy (Morrey and Peterson, 1975), but others recommend a minimum of 3 to 4 weeks parenteral therapy (Blockley and McAllister, 1972; Boland, 1972; Dich et al., 1975; Howard and Nelson, 1976). A recent retrospective study in children with *S. aureus* osteomyelitis (Dich et al., 1975), found that 19 % of those treated with parenteral antibiotics for less than 3 weeks had recurrent or chronic disease, as compared with only 2 % of those treated parenterally for more than 3 weeks. Until an adequately controlled, large scale, prospective study has been carried out in which the short and long term results of various regimens are compared, we continue to recommend at least 3 weeks of appropriate IV antibiotics.

1.4.4 Monitoring of Therapy

When circumstances make this regimen impractical, serum bacteriostatic and bactericidal activity against the patient's organism should be determined in the laboratory. Blood is drawn immediately before a dose of the drug, and again at the time of calculated peak activity (usually 10 to 15 minutes following IV infusion, and 1 to 2 hours following oral doses), first with the clinically adequate IV dose and subsequently with the proposed oral dose. Preliminary experience suggests a correlation between successful outcome and peak bactericidal titres of at least 1:8. Theoretically, antibiotic concentrations in bone should be of primary importance, but methodological problems and insufficient data limit their clinical relevance (Kolczun et al., 1974; Norden, 1971; Parsons, 1976; Smilack et al., 1976).

1.4.5 Surgical Treatment

The timing and extent of surgical intervention are controversial (Blockley and McAllister, 1972; Boland, 1972; Morrey and Peterson, 1975; Waldvogel et al., 1970). Antibiotics alone are usually fully effective in cases where therapy is begun before bone changes are radiographically demonstrable. We feel that surgery is usually warranted when there is evidence of bone destruction or accumulation of pus; puncture wounds, foreign bodies and major open trauma generally demand at least debridement (Fitzgerald et al., 1975; Waldvogel et al., 1970). Continuous or intermittent suction-irrigation of the debrided bone may be useful (Boland, 1972; Lawyer and Eyring, 1972).

Immobilisation may be necessary for pain relief and prevention of pathological fracture. Subacute and chronic osteomyelitis are ordinarily managed surgically, with antibiotic therapy (frequently of long duration) playing an important but perhaps adjunctive role (Chater et al., 1972; Hedstrom, 1975; Rowling, 1970; Waldvogel et al., 1970).

2. Septic Arthritis

Childhood septic arthritis is most often associated with bacteraemia and a focus of infection elsewhere in the body; less commonly it is a complication of osteomyelitis in an adjacent bone. Even with antibiotic use, potentially crippling sequelae are seen, especially with pyarthrosis of the hip (Howard et al., 1976).

2.1 Aetiology

Staphylococcus aureus, Haemophilus influenzae and various streptococci together account for the vast majority of cases of septic arthritis (Morrey ct al., 1975; Nelson, 1972). *H. influenzae* is more common in infants under the age of 2 to 3 years, and *S. aureus* in older children. Other pathogens such as gonococci, meningococci and pneumococci make up a smaller but still significant proportion. Enteric Gram-negative bacilli are also encountered, as well as various other organisms such as anaerobes and fungi.

Pyarthrosis in neonates may reflect the environment associated with the intensive care nursery (Pittard et al., 1976). Tuberculous arthritis is uncommon today but may be seen in cases of widespread disease.

2.2 Clinical Features

Children with septic arthritis frequently present with fever, irritability and guarding of the involved joint. Careful physical examination usually reveals characteristic signs of joint pain and swelling. Unlike that with sterile 'sympathetic' effusions associated with osteomyelitis, pain in pyarthrosis is exacerbated by passive motion of or increased pressure in the joint. Associated signs of inflammation, such as leucocytosis with a left shift and an elevated erythrocyte sedimentation rate, may be

present but are not reliably found. Plain radiograms may show joint capsule distension, obliteration of periarticular soft tissue planes, or vicinal osteomyelitis.

2.3 Diagnosis

The principal diagnostic tool is arthrocentesis with careful analysis of the fluid.
Gram stain often reveals abundant polymorphonuclear leucocytes, and the responsible bacteria may be directly visualised. Joint fluid protein is usually elevated,
and glucose concentration may be low or normal. The fluid should be immediately
cultured in a relatively large volume of the appropriate nutrient broth, because
purulent fluid is an unfavourable environment for bacterial survival. Blood cultures
should be taken before and after the arthrocentesis. Any associated infection, such as
pharyngitis, conjunctivitis, vaginitis, urethritis or meningitis must also be evaluated
with appropriate specimens taken for Gram stain and culture.

Because of the importance of relatively fastidious organisms such as *H. influenzae* and pathogenic neisseriae, the clinician should make certain that cultures are set
up without delay on especially supportive media such as chocolate or Levinthal's agar
in addition to the routine media, and incubated in a CO_2-enriched atmosphere. Newer
techniques such as counterimmunoelectrophoresis (CIE) have shown promise in the
rapid diagnosis of bacteraemic infections due to *H. influenzae*; although the use of
CIE in the evaluation of septic arthritis has been proposed (Merritt et al., 1976), it remains to be shown useful.

The role of radionuclide scanning in early diagnosis remains to be defined,
although [67]gallium citrate may show asymmetry consistent with local inflammation.

2.4 Treatment

2.4.1 Initial Therapy

If the Gram stain of joint fluid reveals polymorphonuclear leucocytes and Gram-
positive cocci, therapy should be initiated with a penicillinase resistant β-lactam antibiotic such as cloxacillin or nafcillin (150 to 200mg/kg/day IV), etc. A cephalosporin
may be acceptable in cases of penicillin allergy. Pleomorphic Gram-negative coccobacilli in a child over the age of 1 month are most likely to be *H. influenzae*,
although neisseriae, moraxellae, etc. may occasionally be difficult to distinguish. In
areas where ampicillin resistant strains of *H. influenzae* are prevalent, chloramphenicol (100mg/kg/day IV) should be given with ampicillin (150mg/kg/day in 4
to 6 divided doses IV) in the initial therapy of septic arthritis in children under age 4
years until diagnostic bacteriology demonstrates the absence of an ampicillin resistant
strain.

In neonates, or in other circumstances where enteric bacterial infection is likely,
initial therapy should include ampicillin plus an aminoglycoside such as kanamycin

Table I. Summary of the treatment of common infections of the skeletal system in infancy and childhood

---

1. *Osteomyelitis*
   a) Accurate bacteriological diagnosis important: cultures of blood, bone lesion and any associated infection
   b) Because of predominance of staphylococci in aetiology, use an antistaphylococcal penicillin e.g. cloxacillin (150 to 200mg/kg/day IV) initially. If necessary, change to more appropriate drug (e.g. penicillin G for *Strep. pyogenes*) when bacteriological identification complete
   c) If Gram-negative rods seen on initial Gram stain, use ampicillin (150 to 200mg/kg/day IV) plus an aminoglycoside (e.g. kanamycin, 20mg/kg/day IM or IV or gentamicin, 5 to 7.5mg/kg/day IM or IV); give gentamicin if *Pseudomonas* suspected (e.g. puncture wound)
   d) In penicillin hypersensitive patients, use a cephalosporin, clindamycin or fusidic acid
   e) Continue IV antibiotic therapy for at least 3 weeks. Where possible, monitor peak serum bacteriostatic and bactericidal activity against patient's organism; a peak bactericidal titre of 1:8 appears to correlate with successful outcome
   f) Surgical intervention warranted if there is evidence of bone destruction or accumulation of pus

2. *Septic arthritis*
   a) Arthrocentesis with careful examination of fluid is principal diagnostic tool
   b) If Gram stain reveals Gram-positive cocci, initiate therapy with antistaphylococcal penicillin (e.g. cloxacillin or nafcillin, 150 to 200mg/kg/day IV); use a cephalosporin or clindamycin in penicillin hypersensitive patients
   c) In children under 4 years of age and where Gram stain reveals pleomorphic Gram-negative coccobacilli (most likely *H. influenzae*), initiate therapy with ampicillin (150mg/kg/day IV); add chloramphenicol (100mg/kg/day IV) in areas where ampicillin resistant strains prevalent
   d) In neonates and where enteric bacterial infection likely, initiate therapy with ampicillin plus an aminoglycoside (e.g. kanamycin, 20mg/kg/day IM or IV or gentamicin, 5 to 7.5mg/kg/day IM or IV)
   e) Continuing therapy guided by sensitivity testing
   f) Continue treatment for at least 2 to 3 weeks; up to 6 weeks in presence of osteomyelitis
   g) Adequate drainage and irrigation necessary with most septic joints; arthrotomy required in pyarthrosis of the hip

---

(20mg/kg/day in 2 to 3 divided doses IM or IV) or gentamicin (5 to 7.5mg/kg/day in 2 to 3 divided IM or IV doses). *Pseudomonas aeruginosa* may be suspected in the case of an infection due to a puncture wound, and in such cases gentamicin should be selected.

2.4.2 Continuing Therapy

Once a bacteriological identification has been made and the organism's sensitivities are known, therapy should be changed (if necessary) to the most active, most specific, best tolerated and least toxic antibiotic. For example, Group A and viridans streptococci, penicillin sensitive staphylococci, pneumococci, gonococci and meningococci should be treated with penicillin G (100,000u/kg/day in 6 divided doses); group B streptococci are slightly less sensitive and should be treated with maximum doses of penicillin G (up to 250,000u/kg/day). Ampicillin sensitive *H. influenzae* should be effectively eradicated with ampicillin; a resistant isolate (defined by an ampicillin MIC > 2μg/ml or the production of β-lactamase) should be treated with chloramphenicol.

Penicillinase producing staphylococci should be treated with a penicillinase resistant antibiotic such as cloxacillin (200mg/kg/day IV in 4 to 6 divided doses) or a cephalosporin (e.g. cephalothin 150mg/kg/day IV). If documented hypersensitivity to both penicillins and cephalosporins exists, a macrolide such as erythromycin or clindamycin may be effective against staphylococci (Feigin, 1975), but arthrocenteses should be repeated to ensure that adequate inhibitory and bactericidal activity are obtained in the joint fluid (Parker and Schmid, 1971).

Although formerly used as an adjunctive therapy, intra-articular administration of antibiotics has been shown to be unnecessary because of good penetration of most antibiotics into the joint cavity (Chow et al., 1971; Nelson, 1971; Parker and Schmid, 1971).

2.4.3 Duration of Therapy

The optimum duration of antibiotic therapy in septic arthritis remains to be determined, but most workers recommend a minimum of 2 to 3 weeks, and up to 6 weeks in the presence of osteomyelitis. The duration of parenteral therapy is also controversial; as discussed above (section 1.4.4), if oral therapy can be shown to provide satisfactory serum inhibitory and bactericidal levels, an outcome comparable to that obtainable with IV therapy should theoretically be expected, although yet to be proved.

2.4.4 Surgical Treatment

Adequate drainage and irrigation (Goldenberg et al., 1975) is necessary in the treatment of most septic joints (with the possible exception of meningococcal and gonococcal arthritis), because of the destructive effects on articular cartilage of pus (due to leucocyte enzymes, bacterial activity and enzymes, pH, etc.) [Daniel et al., 1976]. After initial aspiration, the joint cavity should be lavaged until the return is clear; if any signs of re-accumulation of effusion are recognised, the process should be repeated as often as necessary. The major exception to this conservative management is pyarthrosis of the hip, which is often a surgical emergency as it has been shown that the eventual prognosis for the joint is inversely correlated with the duration of symptoms (Weisgerber et al., 1973). By virtue of its anatomy, with blood supply to the femoral head traversing a joint cavity surrounded by a relatively non-distensible capsule, the hip joint is especially susceptible to irreversible major damage by infarction due to increased intra-articular pressure caused by the accumulation of pus: many workers therefore recommend immediate arthrotomy of the septic hip (Howard et al., 1976; Morrey et al., 1976; Weisgerber et al., 1973).

3. Other Infections

Other, less common, infections of the skeletal system in children will not be reviewed here. For discussions of infections of the intervertebral disc space readers are referred to specific reviews on this subject (Boston et al., 1975; Lascari et al., 1967; Rocco and Eyring, 1972); vertebral body osteomyelitis is primarily a disease of adults, in part related to anatomical differences (Musher et al., 1976; Stauffer, 1975). Osteomyelitis associated with animal bites, occasionally involving organisms such as *Pasteurella multocida,* has been discussed by Szalay and Sommerstein (1972) and others (Griffin and Barber, 1975; Szalay, 1975; Tee, 1975).

Bone infections caused by fungi, mycobacteria, etc., have been reviewed by Edwards et al. (1975), Hirschmann and Everett (1976) and Pritchard (1975).

4. Conclusions

Infections of the skeletal system remain a major diagnostic and therapeutic problem, despite the continuing evolution of techniques and antimicrobial agents. Aggressive approaches to diagnosis, utilisation of the best microbiological and radiological methods, rational selection of antibiotics, judicious surgical intervention when appropriate, and avoidance of overly brief courses of antibiotic therapy, are among the keys to acceptable results.

References

Barrett-Connor, E.: Bacterial infection and sickle cell anemia. An analysis of 250 infections in 166 patients and a review of the literature. Medicine 50: 97-112 (1971).

Blockey, N.J. and McAllister, T.A.: Antibiotics in acute osteomyelitis in children. Journal of Bone and Joint Surgery (Britain) 54B: 299-309 (1972).

Boland, A.L.: Acute hematogenous osteomyelitis. Orthopedic Clinics of North America 3: 225-239 (1972).

Boston, H.C., Jr.; Bianco, A.J., Jr. and Rodes, K.H.: Disk space infections in children. Orthopedic Clinics of North America 6: 953-964 (1975).

Brand, R.A. and Black, H.: Pseudomonas osteomyelitis puncture wounds in children. Journal of Bone and Joint Surgery (America) 56A: 1637-1642 (1974).

Capitanio, M.A. and Kirkpatrick, J.A.: Early roentgen observation in acute osteomyelitis. American Journal of Roentgenology 108: 488-496 (1970).

Chater, E.H.; Flynn, J. and Wilson, A.L.: Fucidin levels in osteomyelitis. Journal of the Irish Medical Association 65: 506-508 (1972).

Chow, A.; Hecht, R. and Winters, R.: Gentamicin and carbenicillin penetration into the septic joint. New England Journal of Medicine 285: 178-191 (1971).

Crane, L.R.; Kapdi, C.C.; Wolfe, J.N.; Silverberg, B.K. and Lerner, A.M.: Xeroradiography in experimental staphylococcal osteomyelitis. Presented to the 15th Interscience Conference on Antimicrobial Agents and Chemotherapy, Washington, DC, September 25th, 1975 (Abstract No. 295).

Daniel, D.; Akeson, W.; Amiel, D.; Ryder, M. and Boyer, J.: Lavage of septic joints in rabbits: Effects of chondrolysis. Journal of Bone and Joint Surgery (America) 58A: 393-395 (1976).

Dich, V.Q.; Nelson, J.D. and Haltalin, K.C.: Osteomyelitis in infants and children. A review of 163 cases. American Journal of Diseases of Children 129: 1273-1278 (1975).

Diggs, L.W.: Bone and joint lesions in sickle-cell disease. Clinical Orthopedics 52: 119-143 (1967).

Edwards, J.E.; Turkel, S.B.; Elder, H.A.; Rand, R.W. and Guze, L.B.: Hematogenous candida osteomyelitis: Report of 3 cases and review of the literature. American Journal of Medicine 59: 89-94 (1975).

Engh, C.A.; Hughes, J.L.; Abrams, R.C. and Bowerman, J.W.: Osteomyelitis in the patient with sickle-cell disease. Diagnosis and management. Journal of Bone and Joint Surgery (America) 53A: 1-15 (1974).

Epidemiological Research Laboratory: Haemophilus bacteremia. British Medical Journal 2: 651 (1976).

Feigin, R.D.; Pickering, L.K.; Anderson, D.; Keeney, R.E. and Shackelford, P.G.: Clindamycin treatment of osteomyelitis and septic arthritis in children. Pediatrics 55: 213-223 (1975).

Fitzgerald, R.H.; Landells, D.G. and Cowan, J.D.E.: Osteomyelitis in children: Comparison of hematogenous and secondary osteomyelitis. Canadian Medical Association Journal 112: 166-169 (1975).

Gilday, D.L. and Paul, D.J.: The differentiation of osteomyelitis and cellulitis in children using a combined blood pool and bone scan (Abstract). Journal of Nuclear Medicine 15: 494 (1974).

Gledhill, R.B.: Subacute osteomyelitis in children. Clinical Orthopedics 96: 57 (1973).

Goldenberg, D.L.; Brandt, K.D.; Cohen, A.S. and Cathcart, E.S.: Treatment of septic arthritis. Comparison of needle aspiration and surgery as initial modes of joint drainage. Arthritis and Rheumatism 18: 83-90 (1975).

Griffin, A.J. and Barber, H.M.: Joint infection by Pasturella multocida. Lancet 1: 1347-1348 (1975).

Handmaker, H. and Leonards, R.: The bone scan in inflammatory osseous disease. Seminars in Nuclear Medicine 6: 95-105 (1976).

Hedstrom, S.A.: Treatment of chronic staphylococcal osteomyelitis with cloxacillin and dicloxacillin — a comparative study in 12 patients. Scandinavian Journal of Infectious Diseases 7: 55-57 (1975).

Hirschmann, J.V. and Everett, E.D.: Candida osteomyelitis: Case report and review of the literature. Journal of Bone and Joint Surgery (America) 58A: 573-575 (1976).

Howard, J.B.; Highgenboten, C.L. and Nelson, J.D.: Residual effects of septic arthritis in infancy and childhood. Journal of the American Medical Association 236: 932 (1976).

Howard, J.B. and Nelson, J.D.: Septic arthritis and osteomyelitis; in Gellis and Kagan (Eds.) Current Pediatric Therapy — 7, pp.423-427 (Saunders, Philadelphia 1976).

Karayalcin, G.; Rosner, F.; Kim, K.Y.; Chandra, P. and Aballi, A.J.: Sickle-cell anemia — clinical manifestations in 100 patients and reviews of the literature. American Journal of Medical Science 269: 51-68 (1975).

Kolczun, M.C.; Nelson, C.L.; McHenry, M.C.; Gavan, T.L. and Pinovich, P.: Antibiotic concentrations in human bone. Journal of Bone and Joint Surgery (America) 56A: 305-310 (1974).

Lascari, A.D.; Graham, M.H. and MacQueen, J.C.: Intervertebral disk infection in children. Journal of Pediatrics 70: 751-757 (1967).

Lawyer, R.B. and Eyring, E.J.: Intermittent closed suction-irrigation treatment of osteomyelitis. Clinical Orthopedics 88: 80-85 (1972).

Letts, R.M.; Afifi, A. and Sutherland, J.B.: Technetium bone scanning as an aid in the diagnosis of atypical acute osteomyelitis in children. Surgery, Gynecology and Obstetrics 140: 899-902 (1975).

Lutzker, L.G.; Koenigsberg, M. and Freeman, L.M.: Focal bone pain: Infection or infarction? Journal of the American Medical Association 235: 425-426 (1976).

McAllister, T.A.: Treatment of osteomyelitis. British Journal of Hospital Medicine 12: 535-542 (1974).

Merritt, K.; Boyle, W.E.; Dye, S.K. and Porter, R.E.: Counter immunoelectrophoresis in the diagnosis of septic arthritis caused by *Hemophilus influenzae*. Journal of Bone and Joint Surgery (America) 58A: 414-415 (1976).

Miller, E.H. and Semian, D.W.: Gram-negative osteomyelitis following puncture wounds of the foot. Journal of Bone and Joint Surgery (America) 57A: 535-537 (1975).

Minnefor, M.I.; Olson, M.I. and Carver, D.H.: Pseudomonas osteomyelitis following puncture wounds of the foot. Pediatrics 47: 598-601 (1971).

Morrey, B.F.; Bianco, A.J. and Rhodes, K.H.: Septic arthritis in children. Orthopedic Clinics of North America 6: 923-934 (1975).

Morrey, B.F.; Bianco, A.J. and Rhodes, K.H.: Suppurative arthritis of the hip in children. Journal of Bone and Joint Surgery (America) 58A; 388-392 (1976).

Morrey, B.F. and Peterson, H.A.: Hematogenous pyogenic osteomyelitis in children. Orthopedic Clinics of North America 6: 935-951 (1975).

Musher, D.M.; Thorsteinsson, S.B.; Minuth, J.M.N. and Luchi, R.J.: Vertebral osteomyelitis; still a diagnostic pitfall. Archives of Internal Medicine 136: 105-110 (1976).

Nelson, J.D.: Antibiotic concentrations in septic joint effusions. New England Journal of Medicine 284: 349-353 (1971).

Nelson, J.D.: The bacterial etiology and antibiotic management of septic arthritis in infants and children. Pediatrics 50: 437-440 (1972).

Norden, C.W.: Experimental osteomyelitis. II. Therapeutic trials and measurement of antibiotic levels in bone. Journal of Infectious Diseases 124: 565-571 (1971).

Ogden, J.A. and Lister, G.: The pathology of neonatal osteomyelitis. Pediatrics 55: 474-478 (1975).

Parker, R.H. and Schmid, F.R.: Antibacterial activity of synovial fluid during therapy of septic arthritis. Arthritis and Rheumatism 14: 96-104 (1971).

Parsons, R.L.: Antibiotics in bone (Leading Article): Journal of Antimicrobial Chemotherapy 2: 228-230 (1976).

Paul, D.J. and Gilday, D.L.: Polyphosphate bone scanning of non-malignant bone disease in children. Journal of the Canadian Association of Radiologists 26: 285-290 (1975).

Pickering, L.K.; O'Connor, D.M.; Anderson, D.; Bairan, A.C.; Feigin, R.D. and Cherry, J.D.: Comparative evaluation of cefazolin and cephalothin in children. Journal of Pediatrics 85: 842-847 (1974).

Pittard, W.B.; Thullen, J.D. and Fanaroff, A.A.: Neonatal septic arthritis. Journal of Pediatrics 88: 621-624 (1976).

Pritchard, D.J.: Granulomatous infections of bones and joints. Orthopedic Clinics of North America 6: 1029-1047 (1975).

Rocco, H.D. and Eyring, E.J.: Intervertebral disk infections in children. American Journal of Diseases of Children 123: 448-451 (1972).

Rowling, D.E.: Further experience in the management of chronic osteomyelitis. Journal of Bone and Joint Surgery (Britain) 52B: 302-307 (1970).

Season, E.H. and Miller, P.R.: Primary subacute pyogenic osteomyelitis in long bones of children. Journal of Pediatric Surgery 11: 347-353 (1976).

Smilack, J.D.; Flittie, W.H. and Williams, T.W., Jr.: Bone concentrations of antimicrobial agents after parenteral administration. Antimicrobial Agents and Chemotherapy 9: 169-171 (1976).

Stauffer, R.N.: Pyogenic vertebral osteomyelitis. Orthopedic Clinics of North America 6: 1015-1027 (1975).

Szalay, G.C.: Joint infection by Pasturella multocida. Lancet 2: 364 (1975).

Szalay, G.C. and Sommerstein, A.: Inoculation osteomyelitis secondary to animal bites. Clinical Pediatrics 11: 687-689 (1972).

Tedesco, F.J.; Barton, R.W. and Alpers, D.H.: Clindamycin-associated colitis: A prospective study. Annals of Internal Medicine 81: 429-433 (1974).

Tee, G.: Joint infection by Pasturella multocida. Lancet 2: 505 (1975).

Treves, S.; Khettry, J.; Broker, F.H.; Wilkinson, R.H. and Watts, H.: Osteomyelitis: Early scintigraphic detection in children. Pediatrics 57: 173-186 (1976).

Van Wingerden, G.I.; Lolans, V. and Jackson, G.G.: Experimental pseudomonas osteomyelitis: Treatment with sisomycin and carbenicillin. Journal of Bone and Joint Surgery (America) 56A: 1452-1458 (1974).

Waldvogel, F.A.; Medoff, G. and Swartz, M.N.: Osteomyelitis: A review of clinical features, therapeutic considerations and unusual aspects. New England Journal of Medicine 282: 198-206; 260-266; and 316-322 (1970).

Weisgerber, G.; Boureau, M. and Bensahel, H.: L'arthrite aigue de la hanche chez le nouveau-ne et le nourisson. Archives Francaises de Pediatrie 30: 83-94 (1973).

Weissberg, E.D.; Smith, A.L. and Smith, D.H.: Clinical features of neonatal osteomyelitis. Pediatrics 53: 505-510 (1974).

Chapter VII

Enteric Infections

M.I. Marks

Approximately one quarter of the cases of gastroenteritis and enterocolitis syndrome in children are caused by bacterial pathogens (Grady and Keusch, 1971a,b; Marks, 1973). This may vary with epidemic and endemic conditions. In certain areas of the world *Vibrio cholerae* (Carpenter and Hirschhorn, 1972), *Vibrio parahaemolyticus* (Peffers and Bailey, 1973), or *Escherichia coli* (Guerrant et al., 1975; Merson et al., 1976) are the predominant bacterial causes of diarrhoea. The quality of drinking water, hygiene and sewage treatment facilities are important, as well as the cultural characteristics of the population in question. The custom of eating raw sea fish, for example, is associated with an increased incidence of *Vibrio parahaemolyticus* gastroenteritis in Japan (Peffers and Bailey, 1973).

1. Salmonella Gastroenteritis and Enteric Fever

Salmonellae are ubiquitous organisms found in many food products, and complex host-parasite relationships are involved in the pathogenesis of, and recovery from, human infection with these bacteria (Maier and Oels, 1972; Venneman and Berry, 1971a,b). These complexities make the prevention, control and therapy of this type of gastroenteritis very difficult.

1.1 Salmonella Gastroenteritis

1.1.1 Pathogenesis and Clinical Features

Salmonellae are common causes of foodborne epidemics and sporadic enterocolitis of children. Histopathologically, there is extensive inflammation of the small and, often, the large intestine with shallow ulceration and superficial necrosis. These are invasive bacteria and bacteraemia is frequently encountered in association with enterocolitis; extragastrointestinal complications in infants and children are serious, *albeit* rare in developed countries.

1.1.2 Treatment

Abnormal host defence mechanisms including defects of humoral immunity, macrophage activity, secretory IgA, cell-mediated immunity and other factors increase the potential for invasiveness and extragastrointestinal complications with Salmonella infection. Children with immunological abnormalities are, therefore, often treated with antibiotics, even though they manifest only the enterocolitis form of infection. For this purpose, ampicillin 100mg/kg/day can be given. Amoxycillin or co-trimoxazole are suitable alternatives.

Parenteral ampicillin in a dosage of 200mg/kg/day is often necessary to treat extragastrointestinal complications. Young infants, leukaemics, hosts with natural or drug induced immunological suppression and debilitated patients with neoplasms should probably receive this type of therapy after careful clinical and laboratory examinations have been carried out to document the presence of extragastrointestinal disease.

The natural course of illness of Salmonella gastroenteritis in children is usually a benign one and the carrier state, as measured by Salmonella excretion in the stools, is not prolonged beyond eight weeks (Kazemi et al., 1973). Under the age of 3 months, this may not be true, as infants may excrete Salmonella in the stools for a period of 2 to 3 months (Kazemi et al., 1973). Efforts to treat enterocolitis with oral antibacterials such as ampicillin or co-trimoxazole have not been successful and, in adults, have been demonstrated to increase the carrier state as well as favour the appearance of bacteria resistant to antibiotic therapy (Kazemi et al., 1974; Schroeder et al., 1968). Additionally, and most importantly, oral antibiotic therapy does not appear to shorten the morbidity or complication rate of gastrointestinal salmonellosis (Kazemi et al., 1974).

1.2 Enteric Fever

Typhoid and paratyphoid fevers are uncommon in developed countries but frequent where malnutrition, poor hygiene, inadequate sewage facilities and parasitic infestations abound.

1.2.1 Pathogenesis and Clinical Features

S. typhi is carried and excreted for any length of time only by man; water is the most important vehicle in the spread of infection. Other *Salmonella* spp. are common in fowl and livestock and spread can be food-borne, animal-mediated or person to person. Salmonellae (*S. typhi, paratyphi* and occasionally other types) colonise the gastrointestinal tract of man after ingestion of contaminated water, food or fomites.

Gastrointestinal signs may include diarrhoea and vomiting in children under 2 years of age, but usually consist of abdominal distension or vague epigastric discomfort. Constipation, headache, cough, tender splenomegaly and fever may be present. Fever, malaise and mild anorexia may be the only features of infection in children and the course of illness is usually less severe than that seen in adults. Thus enteric fever in children may present as:

1) Acute toxaemia (severe cases may be present with septic shock).

2) Prolonged febrile illness with abdominal pain, splenomegaly, anorexia and fever.

3) Diarrhoea, vomiting, meningitis and high fever in patients under 2 years of age.

The second type of presentation may escape diagnosis in developed countries and remit and recur over weeks or months (often presenting as a 'fever of unknown origin' syndrome). Any of these forms may occur in combination with Shigella infections or schistosomiasis (Farid et al., 1975; Kamat and Herzog, 1977). Acute and chronic forms of urinary tract infections may be encountered when Salmonella infection occurs together with, or superimposed upon, *S. haematobium* infection. Chronic carriage and excretion of Salmonella after enteric fever is much less frequent in children (2 to 3 %) than in adults.

1.2.2 Diagnosis

The diagnosis of enteric fever depends upon culture of Salmonella from the blood, urine and/or stool. Serological diagnosis in individual cases is unreliable as paired sera are usually not available and lack of specificity makes interpretation of results difficult.

1.2.3 Treatment

Treatment of enteric fever begins with antibacterial therapy and should, thereafter, include recommendations for isolation of the patient, treatment of fomites, investigation and management of contacts and the source of infection. Of course, the child in shock (hypotension, tachycardia, disorientation, hyper- or hypopyrexia, etc.) should be treated immediately with intravenous fluids and corticosteroids in addition to antibacterial therapy.

Several antibacterials are of proven usefulness in enteric fever (Herzog, 1976; Butler et al., 1977). These include chloramphenicol (50 to 100mg/kg/day), ampicillin (100 to 200mg/kg/day), amoxycillin (100mg/kg/day) and co-trimoxazole (10mg trimethoprim/50mg sulphamethoxazole/kg/day). All are administered in 4 divided doses, except for co-trimoxazole which is given twice daily. Meningitis, abscesses and osteomyelitis should be treated with the highest recommended dosages.

There is no one drug that can be relied upon in all cases. Chloramphenicol can precipitate toxaemia and may be associated with a higher relapse rate; however, rapid defervescence (3 to 5 days) and resolution of symptoms is usually the rule with chloramphenicol. The use of this inexpensive drug is limited in many countries now because of the presence of chloramphenicol resistance in many strains of Salmonella. For example, as many as 80 % of *S. typhi* isolated in the Far East are resistant to chloramphenicol. This is also a major problem in Mexico and parts of Africa (Herzog, 1976; Butler et al., 1977). Chloramphenicol is contraindicated in children with glucose-6-phosphate dehydrogenase (G6PD) deficiency and its use carries the well known risk of other haematological complications. Those adverse effects that are dose related are common as many authorities recommend antibacterial therapy in enteric fever for 14 to 21 days. Chloramphenicol serum concentrations are erratic and often suboptimal when the drug is administered intramuscularly.

Ampicillin has an excellent record in the treatment of milder, more chronic enteric fevers (Butler et al., 1977), although it carries a small risk of failure in the acute fulminant illness. Amoxycillin is better absorbed from the gastrointestinal tract and, although experience with this drug is limited, it may be associated with less failures and relapses than ampicillin (Scragg, 1976). Amoxycillin is also very useful in the treatment of carriers. Chloramphenicol resistant strains may also be resistant to ampicillin/amoxycillin, however, and laboratory confirmation of sensitivities should be obtained.

Co-trimoxazole is a most useful drug for enteric fever and is active against most chloramphenicol and ampicillin resistant strains (Herzog, 1976; Butler et al., 1977). Failures, relapses and chronic carriage are uncommon with co-trimoxazole but experience is relatively recent and often poorly controlled. G6PD deficiency is a contraindication to its use.

The complexities of therapeutics in children with enteric fever, combined infections and predisposing conditions are beyond the scope of this book. The answers lie not in vaccine usage (typhoid and paratyphoid vaccines are available but have a poor record for control of endemic disease), but in community-orientated programmes designed to improve hygiene, water supply, sewage facilities and nutritional standards.

2. Yersinia Enterocolitis

2.1 Pathogenesis and Clinical Features

Yersinia enterocolitica is becoming recognised as a major bacterial pathogen of gastroenteritis in children (Kohl et al., 1976; Nilehn, 1969). Young children (usually under 5 years of age) manifest infection by a febrile gastroenteritis syndrome including vomiting and diarrhoea, with or without abdominal pain. This disease is usually benign and self limiting. Older children often manifest a more severe disease with marked abdominal pain and an appendicitis-like syndrome. It is unclear whether antibiotics shorten the course of illness in either of these two syndromes.

Although the epidemiology of Yersinia enterocolitis is incompletely understood, more than 5000 cases have been reported during the last decade (Toma and Deidrick, 1976). Special techniques for laboratory isolation include cold enrichment (taking advantage of the capacity of these bacteria to multiply at room and refrigerator temperature) [Greenwood et al., 1975]. *Yersinia enterocolitica* has been found in drinking water and many domestic animals (Toma and Deidrick, 1975). Many laboratory, epidemiological and pathophysiological features are shared by Yersinia and Salmonella enterocolitis.

2.2 Treatment

Control of disease due to these bacteria on a community basis will depend on strict hygienic measures, isolation procedures and food surveillance rather than specific antibiotic therapy. *Yersinia enterocolitica* is often resistant to ampicillin *in vitro*, but most strains appear to be inhibited by co-trimoxazole or tetracycline (Hammerberg et al., 1977). Clinical trials are insufficient to justify antibiotic therapy for all infected individuals.

3. Shigellosis

3.1 Pathogenesis and Clinical Features

Shigellae cause dysentery-type enterocolitis in children by direct invasion and ulcer formation in the small and large bowel (Keusch et al., 1976). Clinical features of Shigella enterocolitis in children include severe abdominal pain, bloody diarrhoea, fever and convulsions (Nelson and Haltalin, 1971).

Vaccine studies have emphasised the importance of adherence, penetration and local antibody in the pathogenesis of this disease (Dupont, 1975). Two candidate vaccines, a streptomycin-dependent and a mutant hybrid bacteria, look promising in early vaccination studies (Dupont, 1975). Prevention of shigellosis in institutions may be possible in the near future; however, the prospects for community application are remote.

3.2 Treatment

Although it is clear that antibiotic therapy is effective in shortening the clinical and bacteriological course of Shigella enterocolitis, the development of antibiotic resistant strains is a limiting factor (Ross et al., 1972). *Shigella sonnei* and *flexneri* have become increasingly resistant to ampicillin in many areas of the world (Byers et al., 1976). Efforts to substitute other antibiotics such as co-trimoxazole have met with success in recent controlled studies (Nelson et al., 1976). Nevertheless, restriction of antibiotic therapy to Shigella enterocolitis in hospitalised patients and/or those who are severely ill or at high risk due to underlying host factors seems reasonable.

As with Salmonella and Yersinia, hygienic techniques, isolation procedures and community application of programmes for food, water and sewage handling, are of paramount importance in the control of disease due to this bacteria. When antibiotic treatment is indicated, ampicillin 100 to 200mg/kg/day orally or parenterally (the latter route should be used for toxic patients and those with extragastrointestinal infection) is preferred if susceptibility studies indicate sensitivity (Haltalin et al., 1968). If resistance to ampicillin is encountered, co-trimoxazole (10mg trimethoprim/50mg sulphamethoxazole/kg/day) should be substituted and laboratory confirmation of susceptibility is indicated.

Five days of therapy is sufficient for gastrointestinal shigellosis; however, infection elsewhere in the body often requires longer therapy.

4. *Escherichia coli* Enterocolitis

Although *E. coli* was formerly thought to be a major cause of gastroenteritis in children, its role in gastrointestinal infections is undergoing reconsideration (Echeverria et al., 1976; Gross et al., 1976).

4.1 Pathogenesis and Clinical Features

Pathogenetic mechanisms described for *E. coli* enterocolitis include the production of enterotoxin (similar to the enterotoxin produced by *Vibrio cholerae* which causes a watery type of diarrhoea) and/or the capacity to invade, leading to a dysentery type of diarrhoea (Gross et al., 1976). Surprisingly, many *E. coli* of the classic serotypes associated with 'enteropathogenicity' in the past do not have the capacity to produce enterotoxin or to invade the mucosal epithelial cells (Echeverria et al., 1976; Gross et al., 1976). Alternatively, enterotoxin producing *E. coli* (often with no serotype marker of 'enteropathogenicity') have been discovered in travellers suffering from watery diarrhoea (Merson et al., 1976).

Table I. Summary of the treatment of common bacterial enteric infections in infancy and childhood

---

1. *Salmonella gastroenteritis*
   a) No treatment necessary in most cases (natural course of illness is usually benign).
   b) In children with immunological abnormalities, treat with ampicillin (100mg/kg/day) orally or parenterally; amoxycillin or co-trimoxazole are suitable alternatives.
   c) If extragastrointestinal disease present, treat with parenteral ampicillin (200mg/kg/day).

2. *Enteric fever*
   a) In acute toxaemic patients, treat shock if present and administer chloramphenicol 100mg/kg/day in 4 divided doses IV. Use ampicillin 200mg/kg/day in patients with G6PD deficiency and in those infected with chloramphenicol resistant strains.
   b) For less severe illness where oral therapy is possible, use amoxycillin 100mg/kg/day or chloramphenicol 50 to 100mg/kg/day, both in 4 divided doses. Co-trimoxazole (10mg tri-methoprim/50mg sulphamethoxazole/kg/day) in 2 divided doses is also useful.
   c) Laboratory confirmation of sensitivity, careful follow-up and hygienic measures are essential.

3. *Yersinia enterocolitis*
   a) Role of antibiotic therapy remains to be defined.
   b) Most strains of *Yersinia enterocolitica* are sensitive to co-trimoxazole or tetracycline, but often resistant to ampicillin.
   c) Control of disease depends more on strict hygiene measures than on specific antibiotic therapy.

4. *Shigellosis*
   a) Antibiotic therapy should be restricted to hospitalised patients and/or those who are severely ill or at risk due to underlying host factors.
   b) When antibiotics indicated, use ampicillin (100 to 200mg/kg/day orally or parenterally); if organism resistant to ampicillin, substitute co-trimoxazole (10mg trimethoprim/50mg sulphamethoxazole/
      kg/day) if susceptibility confirmed.
   c) 5 days of therapy is usually sufficient.

5. E. coli *enterocolitis*
   a) Antibiotic therapy used only as an adjunct to other control measures.
   b) Use of neomycin (100mg/kg/day) or colistin (10 to 15mg/kg/day) for 3 days produces clinical improvement and decreased bacterial excretion.
   c) Therapy of enterotoxin producing *E. coli* disease is probably limited to hygiene, isolation, fluid and electrolyte therapy.

4.2 Treatment

Antibiotic therapy of invasive *E. coli* disease has not been studied well enough to suggest a single approach. Use of an oral aminoglycoside or polypeptide (such as neomycin 100mg/kg/day or colistin 10 to 15mg/kg/day in divided doses) for three days is attended by clinical improvement, decreased bacterial excretion and a minimal risk of antibiotic induced diarrhoea (Nelson, 1971). The therapy of enterotoxin producing *E. coli* disease is probably limited to hygiene, isolation, fluid and electrolyte therapy.

5. Gastroenteritis due to Other Bacteria

As mentioned above, *Vibrio parahaemolyticus* is an important cause of foodborne gastroenteritis in countries in which uncooked seafood is ingested (Peffers and Bailey, 1973). Special laboratory techniques are necessary to recognise this bacteria. Cholera is still ubiquitous, and its control requires general hygienic and sanitation approaches (Carpenter, 1971; Carpenter and Hirschhorn, 1972). Although antibiotic therapy (e.g. with tetracycline or chloramphenicol) is effective in reducing shedding of *Vibrio cholerae* in the stools, it is only adjunctive to fluid and electrolyte management.

Staphylococcus aureus occasionally causes severe enterocolitis; however, it is a rare pathogen in the normal host. Similarly, other organisms such as Proteus, *Clostridium perfringens*, Klebsiella, etc. are implicated in certain foodborne outbreaks but their role in the causation of gastroenteritis and enterocolitis in other circumstances is poorly defined. The isolation in the laboratory of these pathogens, as well as Pseudomonas and various other bacteria is by no means proof of their causative role in patients with diarrhoea. This is particularly important as antimicrobial therapy of these bacteria require toxic medications which introduce unnecessary hazards to the patient.

6. General Aspects of Treatment

In general, antibiotic therapy of bacterial gastroenteritis in children is restricted to severe and protracted disease and/or disease in which extragastrointestinal complications are apparent or suspected. The role of antibiotic therapy in the treatment of Shigella and *Yersinia enterocolitica* infection remains to be defined. Antibiotic therapy in *Escherichia coli* and cholera infections is usually only adjunctive to other control measures. The choice of antibiotics should depend on resistance patterns in the specific community and confirmation by *in vitro* susceptibility testing in the diagnostic microbiology laboratory. Strict handwashing is the most important method of preventing spread of enteric infection in the family, hospital and community. Fluid and electrolyte therapy is important, especially for those diseases due to enterotoxin producing bacteria.

Antimotility agents such as diphenoxylate/atropine ('Lomotil') and others can be dangerous in children, and their use is contraindicated (Medical Letter, 1975; Novak et al., 1976). Similarly, the risks of clioquinol (iodochlorhydroxyquin) do not warrant its use either prophylactically or therapeutically in gastroenteritis in children. Other agents such as *Lactobacillus acidophilus,* or kaolin/pectin suspensions have been shown not to be effective in recent clinical trials (Pearce and Hamilton, 1974; Portnoy et al., 1975). Further studies are indicated to define the pathogenesis of diarrhoea in the majority of children and the possible interactions of bacteria with other causes of gastroenteritis. Controlled clinical studies are also warranted to better evaluate the use of antibiotic therapy in newly recognised bacterial pathogens of children such as *Yersinia enterocolitica,* and in *E. coli* enterocolitis relevant to recently discovered pathogenetic mechanisms.

References

Butler, T.; Linh, N.N.; Arnold, K.; Adickman, M.D.; Chau, D.M. and Muoi, M.M.: Therapy of anti-microbial-resistant typhoid fever. Antimicrobial Agents and Chemotherapy 11: 645 (1977).

Byers, P.A.; Dupont, H.L. and Goldschmidt, M.C.: Antimicrobial susceptibilities of shigellae isolated in Houston, Texas, in 1974. Antimicrobial Agents and Chemotherapy 9: 288 (1976).

Carpenter, C.C.J., Jr.: Cholera enterotoxin — recent investigations yield insights into transport processes. American Journal of Medicine 50: 1 (1971).

Carpenter, C.C.J., Jr. and Hirschhorn, N.: Pediatric cholera: Current concepts of therapy. Tropical Pediatrics 80: 874 (1972).

Dupont, H.L.: Recent developments in immunization against diarrheal disease. Southern Medical Journal 68: 1027 (1975).

Echeverria, P.D.; Chang, C.P. and Smith, D.: Enterotoxigenicity and invasive capacity of 'enteropathogenic' serotypes of *Escherichia coli.* Journal of Pediatrics 89: 8 (1976).

Farid, Z.; Miner, W.F. and Hassan, A.: Enteric fever in Egypt. Medical Progress 2(No. 2): 23 (Feb. 1975).

Grady, G.F. and Keusch, G.T.: Pathogenesis of bacterial diarrheas. I. New England Journal of Medicine 285: 831 (1971a).

Grady, G.F. and Keusch, G.T.: Pathogenesis of bacterial diarrheas. II. New England Journal of Medicine 285: 891 (1971b).

Greenwood, J.R.; Flanigan, S.M.; Pickett, M.D. and Martin, W.J.: Clinical isolation of *Yersinia enterocolitica:* Cold temperature enrichment. Journal of Clinical Microbiology 2: 559 (1975).

Gross, R.J.; Scotland, S.M. and Rowe, B.: Enterotoxin testing of *Escherichia coli* causing epidemic infantile enteritis in the U.K. Lancet 1: 629 (1976).

Guerrant, R.L.; Moore, R.A.; Kirschenfeld, P.M. and Sande, M.A.: Role of toxigenic and invasive bacteria in acute diarrhea of childhood. New England Journal of Medicine 293: 567 (1975).

Haltalin, K.C.; Nelson, J.D.; Kusmiesz, H.T. and Hinton, L.V.: Comparison of intramuscular and oral ampicillin therapy for shigellosis. Journal of Pediatrics 73: 617 (1968).

Hammerberg, S.; Sorger, S. and Marks, M.I.: Antimicrobial susceptibilities of *Yersinia enterocolitica* biotype 4, serotype 0:3. Antimicrobial Agents and Chemotherapy 11: 566 (1977).

Herzog, C.: Chemotherapy of typhoid fever: A review of literature. Infection 4: 166 (1976).

Kamat, S.A. and Herzog, C.: Typhoid: Clinical picture and response to chloramphenicol. Infection 5: 85 (1977).

Kazemi, M.; Gumpert, T.G. and Marks, M.I.: A controlled trial of sulfamethoxazole-trimethoprim, ampicillin, or no therapy in the treatment of salmonella gastroenteritis in children. Journal of Pediatrics 83: 646 (1973).

Kazemi, M.; Gumpert, T.G. and Marks, M.I.: The clinical spectrum and carrier state of non-typhoidal salmonella infections in infants and children. I. Canadian Medical Association Journal 110: 1253 (1974).

Keusch, G.T.; Jacewicz, M.; Levine, M.M.; Hornick, R.B. and Kochwa, S.: Pathogenesis of shigella diarrhea. Journal of Clinical Investigation 57: 194 (1976).

Kohl, S.; Jacobson, J.A. and Nahmias, A.: Yersinia enterocolitica in children. Journal of Pediatrics 89: 77 (1976).

Maier, T. and Oels, H.C.: Role of the macrophage in natural resistance to salmonellosis in mice. Infection and Immunity 6: 438 (1972).

Marks, M.I.: The pathogenesis and therapy of Gram-negative bacterial gastroenteritis; in Current Concepts in the Management of Gram-negative Bacterial Infections, Excerpta Medica International Congress Series No.318, p.9 (Excerpta Medica, Amsterdam 1973).

Medical Letter: Lomotil for diarrhea in children. Medical Letter 7: 101 (December, 1975).

Merson, M.H.; Morris, G.K.; Sack, D.A.; Wells, J.G.; Feeley, J.C.; Sack, R.B.; Creech, W.B.; Kapikian, A.Z. and Gangarosa, E.J.: Travelers' diarrhea in Mexico. New England Journal of Medicine 294: 1299 (1976).

Nelson, J.D. and Haltalin, K.C.: Accuracy of diagnosis of bacterial diarrheal disease by clinical features. Journal of Pediatrics 78: 519 (1971).

Nelson, J.D.: Duration of neomycin therapy for enteropathogenic Escherichia coli diarrheal disease: A comparative study of 113 cases. Pediatrics 48: 248 (1971).

Nelson, J.D.; Kusmiesz, H.; Jackson, L.H. and Woodman, E.: Trimethoprim-sulfamethoxazole therapy for shigellosis. Journal of the American Medical Association 235: 1239 (1976).

Nilehn, E.: Studies of Yersinia enterocolitica with special reference to bacterial diagnosis and occurrence in human acute enteric disease. Acta Pathologica et Microbiologica Scandinavica 206(Suppl.): 5 (1969).

Novak, E.; Lee, J.G.; Seckman, C.E.; Phillips, J.P. and DiSanto, A.R.: Unfavourable effect of atropine-diphenoxylate (Lomotil) therapy in lincomycin-caused diarrhea. Journal of the American Medical Association 235: 1451 (1976).

Pearce, J.L. and Hamilton, J.R.: Controlled trial of orally administered lactobacilli in acute infantile diarrhea. Journal of Pediatrics 84: 261 (1974).

Peffers, A.S.R. and Bailey, J.: Vibrio parahaemolyticus gastroenteritis and international air travel. Lancet 1: 143 (1973).

Portnoy, B.L.; Pruitt, D.; Rodriguez, J.T.; Abdo, J.A. and DuPont, H.L.: Efficacy of anti-diarrheal agents in the treatment of acute diarrhea in children. Clinical Research 23: 29A (1975).

Ross, S.; Controni, G. and Khan, W.: Resistance of shigellae to ampicillin and other antibiotics. Its clinical and epidemiological implications. Journal of the American Medical Association 221: 45 (1972).

Schroeder, S.A.; Terry, P.M. and Bennett, J.V.: Antibiotic resistance and transfer factor in salmonella, United States 1967. Journal of the American Medical Association 205: 903 (1968).

Scragg, J.N.: Further experience with amoxycillin in typhoid fever in children. British Medical Journal 2: 1031 (1976).

Toma, S. and Deidrick, V.R.: Isolation of Yersinia enterocolitica from swine. Journal of Clinical Microbiology 2: 478 (1975).

Toma, S. and Deidrick, V.R.: Incidence of Yersinia enterocolitica and Y. pseudotuberculosis infections in Canada, 1975; semiannual report. Canadian Medical Association Journal 114: 16 (1976).

Venneman, M.R. and Berry, L.J.: Serum-mediated resistance induced with immunogenic preparations of Salmonella typhimurium. Infection and Immunity 4: 374 (1971a).

Venneman, M.R. and Berry, L.J.: Cell-mediated resistance induced with immunogenic preparations of Salmonella typhimurium. Infections and Immunity 4: 381 (1971b).

Chapter VIII

Neonatal Infections

H.C. Spratt

Experimental evidence suggests that neonatal host defences are at best immature in comparison with those of older infants and children. Comparative studies of non-specific immune systems have indicated relative deficiencies in polymorphonuclear chemotaxis, opsonisation of certain bacteria, complement/properdin activity and splenic trapping capacity (Gotoff, 1974). Recent data also suggest that leucocyte intracellular bactericidal activity may be deficient in stressed neonates (Wright et al., 1975).

Cell mediated immune systems are operative in the second trimester. Unless abnormally stimulated *in utero*, cord blood concentrations of IgM, IgE and IgA are minimal. Neonatal IgG is largely obtained by materno-fetal transfer, active in the third trimester. Thus an infant born before 34 weeks gestation may be relatively deficient in immunoglobulin. Also, the half-life of transferred IgG is estimated at approximately 23 days and during early infancy, serum concentrations of immunoglobulin fall and may not approach adult levels until 2 years of age. The significance of this physiological hypogammaglobulinaemia is unclear.

Colostral immunoglobulin may be partially absorbed by the human infant, and a protective role has been invoked in neonatal infections and necrotising enterocolitis, perhaps related to secretory IgA activity (Iyengar and Selvaray, 1972; Goldman and Wayne Smith, 1973; Barlow et al., 1974; Stoliar et al., 1976). Some properties of colostral leucocytes have been studied *in vitro*, but their role in breast fed infants is largely unexplored (Goldman and Wayne Smith, 1973).

1. Factors Predisposing to Neonatal Infections

Predisposing factors are recognised in the majority of cases of neonatal infection. The importance of their attempted control cannot be overstated. The list includes:

1) Maternal infection

2) Premature delivery

3) Prolonged rupture of the membranes[1]

4) Prolonged labour with or without birth trauma

5) Perinatal asphyxia with or without birth trauma

6) Coexisting illness (including jaundice)

7) Use of respirators, catheters, monitoring devices, etc.

8) Nursery overcrowding, under ventilation, under staffing and poor sterile technique.

2. Pathogenic Organisms

2.1 Gram-negative Bacteria

Traditional teaching has emphasised the prevalence of Gram-negative organisms in invasive neonatal infection. These include *E. coli, Klebsiella, Enterobacter, Pseudomonas* and *Proteus* species in approximate descending order of prevalence.

2.2 Gram-positive Bacteria

Group B β-haemolytic streptococci also play a major role, accounting for the majority of systemic infections in many nurseries (Feigin, 1976). Two clinical syndromes have been recognised: early onset (less than 10 days of age), and late onset disease (10 days to 4 months of age) [Baker et al., 1973]. Early onset disease is often manifest within hours of birth, with respiratory distress and septicaemic shock as prominent findings, although Howard and McCracken (1974) have described several less classical presentations. Mortality is commonly greater than 50%.

Late onset disease usually results in meningitis, often without documented septicaemia. Most infants survive, but may not escape neurological sequelae. The problems of therapy and clinical relapse were recently discussed in a series of articles by Broughton et al. (1976). Penicillin G 150,000 to 250,000u/kg/day IV is recommended (McCracken, 1976).

Coagulase positive staphylococcal infections are uncommon in current practice, possibly due to improved skin care of the newborn. *Listeria monocytogenes* is an uncommon but serious pathogen, often lethal in early onset disease (Ray and Wedgewood, 1964).

---

1   Prophylactic antibiotics administered to either the mother or infant have not been shown to be effective (Gunn et al., 1970).

3. Principles of Management

Suspicion of infection is founded upon a detailed history of gestational and perinatal events, and a consideration of likely predisposing factors. The value of smear and culture of amniotic fluid, infant gastric contents, and external ear aspirates have been reported by some authors (Blanc, 1961; Scanlon, 1972). Confirmation of systemic bacterial infection relies on Gram's stain and culture of urine, blood and cerebrospinal fluid. Early cases of meningitis or urinary infection may lack evidence of an inflammatory response.

3.1 Choice of Initial Antibiotic Therapy

The choice of initial antibiotic therapy is based upon evaluation of Gram stained material, consideration of the likely pathogens and knowledge of the antibiotic susceptibility profile of potential pathogens in the nursery environment. Ampicillin and gentamicin continue to serve well in most cases, but the emergence of gentamicin resistance amongst *Pseudomonas* species may indicate preference for an alternative aminoglycoside (e.g. amikacin or tobramycin). Therapy should also include careful attention to supportive measures, i.e.:

1. Fluid, electrolyte, acid-base and thermal balance.

2. Cardiorespiratory support, including small fresh whole blood transfusions as required. Early treatment of shock.

3. Isolation of the patient, sterile nursing technique and frequent change of respirator tubing, incubator reservoir fluid, etc.

It should be noted that inappropriate antidiuretic hormone (ADH) secretion may complicate septicaemia and/or meningitis. Oral nystatin may reduce alimentary colonisation with yeasts and perhaps offer prophylaxis against invasive disease.

3.2 Continuing Therapy

Continuing therapy is guided by the clinical response, and serial smear and culture of the infected material. Determination of the minimum inhibitory concentrations (MIC) of the selected antibacterial drugs against the patient's isolate, and the ability of the patient's serum, urine or CSF (as appropriate) to inhibit a standard inoculum of that same isolate are useful. Based on the available data a peak inhibitory power of at least 1:8 dilution is recommended as being satisfactory (Jawetz, 1962; Klastersky et al., 1974). Therapy should continue for a minimum of 14 days in cases of septicaemia, and 21 days in meningitis.

The selection of antibacterial agent, dosage and route of administration is critical. Table I presents a selected guide to their usage.

Table I. Guide to the use of antibacterial drugs in the neonatal period

Antibacterial drug	Dose and route	Comments
Amikacin	15mg/kg/day divided q12h for 1st week of life, then 22.5mg/kg/day divided q8h IV or IM	Pharmacology similar to kanamycin
Ampicillin	50 to 100mg/kg/day divided q12h for 1st week, then 150 to 200mg/kg/day divided q6 to 8h IM/IV	Contains 3.4mmol Na$^+$/g May alter urinary amino acid chromatogram Effective against most streptococci, Listeria, some Gram-negative bacteria
Carbenicillin	*Infants less than 2kg:* 225mg/kg/day divided q8h for 1st week *Infants more than 2kg:* 300mg/kg/day divided q6h for 1st 4 days Thereafter, 400mg/kg/day divided q6h IV	Contains 4.7mmol Na$^+$/g Peak serum levels, 200µg/ml Resistance may develop if used alone. Recommended against *Pseudomonas* and indole-positive *Proteus* species, in combination with an aminoglycoside
Cephalothin	50 to 100mg/kg/day divided q12h for 1st week, then q8h IV	With kanamycin may be effective against methicillin resistant staphylococci, or resistant *E. coli* Very poor CSF penetration
Chloramphenicol	*Infants less than 2kg: also infants more than 2kg but less than 2 weeks old:* 25mg/kg/day in 1 daily dose IV *Infants more than 2 weeks old:* 50mg/kg/day divided q12h IV	Vasomotor collapse (grey baby syndrome) has been reported at 50mg/kg/day Bone marrow toxicity Haemolytic risk in G6PD deficiency Good brain and CSF penetration Monitor blood levels
Cloxacillin	100 to 200mg/kg/day divided q6 to 8h IM/IV	Recommended for penicillinase producing *S. aureus* Toxicity similar to other penicillins

Drug	Dose	Comments
Gentamicin	5mg/kg/day divided q12h for 1st week, then 7.5mg/kg/day divided q12h IM/IV	IV slowly (30 to 60 minutes) Ototoxic;? nephrotoxic May be synergistic with penicillins against Gram-negative bacteria
Kanamycin	*Infants less than 2kg:* 15mg/kg/day divided q12h for 1st week, then 20mg/kg/day divided q12h IM/IV *Infants more than 2kg:* 20mg/kg/day divided q12h for 1st week, then 30mg/kg/day divided q8h IM/IV	Toxicity and use as per gentamicin May be synergistic with penicillins against enteric bacilli, enterococcus and Listeria
Methicillin	*Infants less than 2 weeks:* 50 to 100mg/kg/day divided q12h in infants 2kg or less and q8h in those more than 2kg IM/IV *Infants more than 2 weeks:* 100 to 200mg/kg/day divided q6h IM/IV	May be nephrotoxic in high doses Significance of lower protein binding is unclear
Penicillin G	50,000 to 100,000u/kg/day divided q12h for 1st 4 days, then q6 to 8h IM/IV 100,000 to 250,000u/kg/day for group B streptococcal disease	1 mega unit contains 1.7mmol of Na^+ or K^+ Smaller total dose q12h preferred in premature infant
Polymyxin B	3 to 4mg/kg/day divided q6h IM/IV	Disc diffusion sensitivity test may be unreliable Diffuses poorly into tissues and CSF Availability of newer aminoglycosides may render this agent obsolete
Tobramycin	5 to 7.5mg/kg/day divided q12h for 1st week, then q8h IM/IV	Toxicity and use as per gentamicin Reserved for gentamicin resistant Pseudomonas infections

4. Septicaemia

Abnormalities commonly associated with neonatal septicaemia are summarised in table II. Incidence is estimated at 1:500 to 1:600 live births; mortality at 13 to 45% (Gotoff and Behrman, 1970).

4.1 Clinical Features and Diagnosis

Intrapartum infection may be acquired from contaminated amniotic fluid, or perhaps more commonly by contact with pathogens in the vaginal and perineal flora (Blanc, 1961). Infection is presumed to result from invasion of the umbilical stump, scalp abrasion or wound, circumcision, or mucosal breach. Post-partum infection is usually acquired by direct human contact, less commonly from contaminated equipment. Occasionally, a developmental anomaly of the urinary tract or central nervous system is associated with local infection and systemic disease.

Laboratory diagnosis depends on a positive blood culture, supplemented by examination and culture of the CSF and bladder tap urine. White blood cell count and sedimentation rate may be useful (Zipursky et al., 1976; Adler and Denton, 1975). Meningitis accompanies one third of cases of septicaemia. A focus of infection can be found in up to one half of cases.

4.2 Treatment

Therapy is guided by the clinical response, repeated blood cultures and specific laboratory data. Thus, tube dilution sensitivity tests and estimation of serum inhibitory powers may be the key to success. The blood culture should be repeated two days after the end of therapy. Where preliminary culture data permit, single agent therapy is usually preferred. In cases of Pseudomonas or Listeria sepsis, combination therapy offers an excellent chance of synergistic activity. (Smith et al., 1969; Moellering et al., 1972) [see table I].

5. Meningitis

Neonatal bacterial meningitis remains an unsolved problem. Attempts to improve the efficacy of conventional antibacterial agents have largely failed, as none combine potency, penetration and freedom from unacceptable toxicity. Group B streptococcal meningitis may be less devastating than Gram-negative infections, but mortality still approximates 20%, with sequelae in a significant minority of survivors (Baker et al., 1973; Barton et al., 1973). By comparison a recent cooperative study of Gram-negative neonatal meningitis reported a mortality of 32%, with sequelae in 36% of survivors up to 4 years later (McCracken and Mize, 1976). Infants of low birth weight were at a significant disadvantage.

5.1 Clinical Features and Diagnosis

Clinical diagnosis is notoriously difficult. The classical signs of meningeal irritation are characteristically absent, and evidence of raised intracranial pressure is often delayed; hence the maxim that consideration of sepsis justifies a lumbar puncture in all cases. CSF abnormalities are often impressive, but may be lacking in early cases. Blood and bladder tap urine cultures, and estimation of the blood/CSF sugar ratio are important.

5.2 Treatment

Antibiotic selection is determined by preliminary laboratory data and experience in the individual nursery. Immediate complications of neonatal meningitis include seizures, vasomotor collapse, respiratory failure, inappropriate ADH syndrome, and disseminated intravascular coagulation. Intermediate complications include ventriculitis, subdural effusion, cerebral abscess, major sinus thrombosis, and early hydrocephalus. Careful studies have shown a favourable prognostic correlation with early sterilisation of the CSF (McCracken, 1972). The laboratory estimation of CSF antibiotic concentration and/or inhibitory power may be helpful. However, recent data suggests that daily lumbar intrathecal injections of 1 mg gentamicin added to a parenteral gentamicin + ampicillin regimen confers no additional benefit in unselected cases of Gram-negative meningitis (McCracken and Mize, 1976).

These considerations do not take account of inoculum size, drug dosage or coincident ventriculitis. Available data suggest that ventriculitis is common, and that the intraventricular route provides superior distribution of drug within the CSF space (Kaiser and McGee, 1975; Salmon, 1972). However, reduction of ventricular size due to cerebral oedema may require a cautious approach to this mode of therapy.

Pending further studies, a reasonable choice is parenteral therapy alone for the first 48 hours (e.g. with a combination of ampicillin and gentamicin). Failing CSF sterilisation, ventricular puncture and antibiotic instillation should be considered. If rejected, daily lumbar intrathecal therapy (e.g. gentamicin 2 to 4mg) may offer an advantage, although this hypothesis is untested.

5.3 Prognosis

The poor prognosis of neonatal meningitis is explained by the nature of the pathogens, limited host defences, delay in diagnosis, the anatomical and physiological factors of neuronal-vascular relationships and CSF flow characteristics in the newborn, the presumed frequency of ventriculitis, and lack of an ideal drug. Pathologically, vasculitis leads to oedema, haemorrhage and infarction. Organisation of the fibrinopurulent exudate may occlude ventricular and subarachnoid communications.

Mortality varies from 18% to over 70%, most deaths occurring within 24 hours of diagnosis (Bell and McCormick, 1975; McCracken, 1972). Estimates of the incidence of sequelae vary from 31% to 73% (McCracken, 1972). In one series, hydrocephalus was documented in 31% of survivors (Lorber and Pickering, 1966). Mental retardation, epilepsy, limb paralyses, cranial nerve palsies, ataxia and behavioural and learning disorders make up the list of major deficits.

6. Pneumonia

Autopsy data suggest that neonatal pneumonia is a contributing factor in up to 30% of perinatal deaths (Barter and Hudson, 1974). Predisposing factors are present in the majority of cases, notably amnionitis, prematurity, respiratory distress syndrome or major surgery.

6.1 Pathogenic Organisms

In early cases, pathogens reflect vaginal flora. Barter and Hudson (1974) documented Gram-negative enteric bacilli in 78% of 222 culture positive fatal cases, mostly *Klebsiella* species, *E. coli* and *Pseudomonas aeruginosa*. Approximately half of these patients had more than one pathogen isolated. In late onset disease, no consistent pattern can be established, presumably due to increased survival with blind therapy of suspected sepsis.

Staphylococcal pneumonia is now uncommon, but its hazards remain unchanged. The impact of early onset group B streptococcal disease must be anticipated, but its similarity to the respiratory distress syndrome, and blind therapy of suspected sepsis may mask its true incidence, reinforcing the need for blood cultures (Vollman et al., 1976).

6.2 Diagnosis

We advocate deep endotracheal aspiration with Gram stain and culture in all suspected cases of neonatal pneumonia. Although percutaneous lung aspiration may provide more exact information, we feel the risks of the procedure preclude its routine use in neonates (Mimica et al., 1971).

6.3 Treatment

Successful management depends on optimal supportive care, with provision of humidified oxygen and respiratory support in addition to specific antibacterial therapy. Abrupt deterioration may signify airway obstruction or pneumothorax. Physiotherapy with gentle airway suction is useful.

7. Enteritis

7.1 Pathogenic Organisms

The discovery of *Rotavirus* enteritis, and its description amongst cases of neonatal diarrhoea, has challenged classic concepts of gastroenteritis causation (Murphy et al., 1975). *Salmonella* and *Shigella* species are undoubted pathogens, but the role of *Yersinia enterocolitica* is largely unexplored.

Innumerable case reports have documented the association of specific serotypes of *E. coli* with sporadic and epidemic diarrhoea. However, inconsistencies in volunteer experiments and epidemiological studies were unexplained until the observation of De et al. (1956) that only patient-derived strains were pathogenic in rabbit ileal loop assays. Extension of this line of research has led to the current concept of enterotoxigenic *E. coli* diarrhoea, independent of serotype. Data from Chicago and Arizona has confirmed enterotoxigenic strains in cases of nursery diarrhoea (Gorbach and Khurana, 1972; Boyer et al., 1975). However, numerous parallel studies in infantile gastroenteritis have failed to provide confirmation (Echeverria et al., 1975; Kapikian et al., 1976; Pai, 1976). In Melbourne, a nursery epidemic of *Rotavirus* enteritis coincided with isolation of three different 'enteropathogenic' serotypes of *E. coli* from study infants. All isolates were toxin negative (Bishop et al., 1976). These discrepant data throw doubt on the classic concept of infantile *E. coli* enteritis, and emphasise the need for clarification. The role of invasive strains of *E. coli* remains largely unexplored.

7.2 Treatment

Attention to fluid, electrolyte, acid-base and nutritional requirements is the basis of clinical management. Salmonella and Shigella infections require systemic antibiotic therapy in the neonatal period and for these, ampicillin is the preferred drug. *E. coli* epidemics may be more easily controlled by the use of short course oral therapy with a non-absorbable agent (e.g. neomycin or colistin), in addition to strict isolation procedures (Nelson, 1971a).

8. Urinary Tract Infections

Epidemiological studies of neonatal urinary tract infection have been hampered by limitations of urine sampling. Incidence approximates 1 to 2% of healthy newborns, with an apparent preponderance of males (Littlewood et al., 1969). This sex difference and early onset of symptoms suggest a haematogenous pathogenesis (Albers et al., 1966). Enteric bacteria predominate (Bergstrom et al., 1972).

8.1 Clinical Features and Diagnosis

Clinical features range from an absence of symptoms to a syndrome of neonatal sepsis (Bergstrom et al., 1972). Feeding problems and jaundice deserve emphasis, and the risk of septicaemia is real. Lincoln and Weinberg (1964) have stressed the likelihood of asymptomatic bacteriuria progressing to overt disease, but spontaneous clearance has been reported (Abbott, 1970). Moreover, the female preponderance amongst older children who present *'de novo'* with chronic pyelonephritis implies that the natural history of uncomplicated neonatal pyelonephritis is uncertain.

Diagnosis is suspected by analysis of clean-catch urine, and confirmed by examination of urine obtained by suprapubic aspiration (Kunin, 1975). Pyuria (> 10 WBC/mm^3) is suspicious (Littlewood, 1971); a urinary colony count $> 100,000$ of a single species of bacteria/ml of clean-catch urine is diagnostic (Braude et al., 1967). Lower counts are considered pathological in urine obtained by suprapubic aspiration.

8.2 Treatment

The choice of antibiotic therapy is governed by laboratory sensitivity testing, which should take account of the anticipated urinary concentration of the active agent. Sulphonamides are contraindicated in the early newborn period and while jaundice persists.

Ampicillin is the agent of choice for initial therapy, and may be combined with kanamycin or gentamicin as an interim precaution against Klebsiella-Enterobacter or Pseudomonas infection, or septicaemia (Garrod and O'Grady, 1972). In uncomplicated infections 2 weeks' therapy appears adequate (Bergstrom et al., 1968, 1972; Kincaid-Smith and Fairley, 1969).

8.3 Prognosis

Prognosis has not been thoroughly evaluated. Recurrence has been documented in up to 25% of cases, usually re-infection within the first year (Bergstom et al., 1972). Progression to chronic pyelonephritis occurs in up to 5% of cases (Bergstom et al., 1972; Saxena et al., 1976). Current opinion favours radiological examination of all patients, based on abnormal findings in up to 50% of cases (Saxena et al., 1976). However, except for cases of obstructive uropathy, there is no clear correlation between early radiological findings and recurrence, chronicity or reflux nephropathy of later childhood (Bergstrom et al., 1972; Saxena et al., 1976).

9. Osteomyelitis

9.1 Clinical Features and Diagnosis

In many ways, neonatal osteomyelitis resembles disease in older children. Most cases result from selective haematogenous infection of the metaphysis, and present with local signs of inflammation without early radiographic changes. *Staphylococcus aureus* continues to be the most common pathogen, and successful therapy depends on timely surgical intervention and prolonged specific parenteral antibiotic therapy. However, there are several important differences: sites of bony infection are often multiple in neonates, spread to the epiphysis with growth plate destruction is common, and contiguous septic arthritis has been noted in a majority of cases (Weissberg et al., 1974).

Systemic toxicity however, is uncommon. Special sites of infection include the skull underlying scalp trauma, and the hip region and calcaneus following blood-letting procedures.

As in older children early diagnosis may be facilitated by isotope scan techniques. In our limited experience, ^{99m}Tc polyphosphate (Usher, 1975) and gallium scans are useful in diagnosis and definition of occult disease. Gallium scans may provide an insight into the state of resolution after clinical signs have subsided.

9.2 Treatment

As many of the local complications are explained on the basis of spontaneous decompression of pus (Ogden and Lister, 1975), neonatal osteomyelitis should be considered a surgical emergency. The optimum duration of antibiotic therapy is uncertain, but clinical experience favours a minimum of 6 weeks. Where available, monitoring of peak serum inhibitory power may permit a controlled changeover to oral therapy once an adequate clinical response has been observed.

10. Septic Arthritis

The paucity of case reports has led to the view that neonatal septic arthritis is rare. Indeed, in a review covering the years 1955 to 1970, Nelson (1972) documented

Table II. Clinical findings suggestive of neonatal sepsis, and differential diagnosis

Clinical findings	Common differential diagnosis
General:	
Fever	Haemorrhage
Hypothermia	Birth trauma
Shock	Perinatal asphyxia
Sclerema	Exposure
	Viral infection
Central nervous system:	
Lethargy	Birth trauma and/or haemorrhage
Hypotonia	Perinatal asphyxia
Irregular respiration	Cerebral malformation
Irritability, tremors, seizures	Familial neuropathy/myopathy
	Meningitis
Apnoea	Encephalitis
Vasomotor instability	
Tense fontanelle	
Respiratory system:	
Tachypnoea	Respiratory distress syndrome
Dyspnoea	Meconium aspiration
Cyanosis	Pneumonia
Apnoea	Atelectasis
	Congenital heart disease
	Metabolic acidosis
	CNS disease
	Cystic fibrosis
Gastrointestinal system:	
Abdominal distension	Intestinal obstruction
Hepatomegaly	Congestive heart failure
Vomiting	Severe haemolytic disease
Diarrhoea	Necrotising enterocolitis
Gastrointestinal	Haemorrhagic disease of the newborn
haemorrhage	
Haematological:	
Jaundice	Severe haemolytic disease
Pallor	Haemorrhage
Splenomegaly	Idiopathic thrombocytopenic purpura
Purpura	
Haemorrhage	Neoplasm
	Viral infection

only 7 neonatal cases amongst a total of 221 childhood cases seen at two Dallas hospitals. However, Pittard et al. (1976) noted 9 cases amongst 545 admissions to a neonatal intensive care unit over the period 1972 to 1974. These data agree with those of Weissberg et al. (1974) and confirm a real increase in incidence directly related to the expansion of neonatal services and improved survival of high-risk infants.

10.1 Clinical Features and Diagnosis

Septic arthritis is a direct complication of septicaemia, with or without contiguous osteomyelitis. Most neonates are ill from other causes; many have undergone umbilical catheterisation. In previously uninfected infants systemic toxicity is often absent. The constraints regarding multiplicity of bony and/or articular sites, and the threat of coexisting non-bony infection (e.g. meningitis) apply to septic arthritis as they do to osteomyelitis.

Clinical and preliminary laboratory assessment must be complete before starting therapy. Blood culture is mandatory before and after joint aspiration, since pus may be bactericidal.

10.2 Treatment

Current experience suggests that *Staphylococcus aureus* remains the most common pathogen, with group B streptococci and Gram-negative enteric bacilli also commonly encountered. Parenteral cloxacillin and gentamicin are recommended as inital therapy. Surgical procedures range from a single diagnostic aspiration to exploration of joints and adjacent metaphyses. Septic arthritis of the hip joint is a special case, and arthrotomy may be the wisest course.

Fortunately, penetration of antibiotics into synovial fluid is excellent and sterilisation of the joint space is usually rapid (Chow et al., 1971; Nelson, 1971b). The optimum duration of therapy is undecided, but a regimen of 3 weeks parenteral followed by 3 weeks oral therapy has been successful (Pittard et al., 1976). Serum inhibitory power may provide a guide to therapy.

10.3 Prognosis

Prognosis probably relates to the timing of diagnosis and the presence of contiguous osteomyelitis. Present data suggests that when the latter is absent, good joint function may be anticipated (Pittard et al., 1976; Weissberg et al., 1974).

11. Congenital Syphilis

11.1 Clinical Features and Diagnosis

Congenital syphilis is always a systemic disease; thus multisystem involvement is an important clinical clue to the diagnosis. The presentation of early disease ranges from an insidious anaemia with failure to thrive, to a florid picture with fever, pneumonia, diffuse osteomyelitis and hepatosplenomegaly. Later presentation tends to be eruptive with diffuse variable rash, mucosal erosions, snuffles, periostitis and osteochondritis. Such lesions are highly infectious. Healing results in scarring and bony deformities.

Late disease is commensurate with adult tertiary syphilis. Hutchison's triad (notched incisors, keratitis and deafness) focuses attention on the distribution of lesions in bone, eye and central nervous system.

The diagnosis is confirmed by dark ground microscopy of material from eruptive lesions, by serology and by examination of the cerebrospinal fluid. Serial reaginic titres are valuable in judging the course and activity of disease, but a treponemal test is necessary for firm diagnosis. Current practice favours the fluorescent treponemal antibody-absorption (FTA-Abs) test. This can be made specific for congenital syphilis by assay of cord blood IgM antibody, and quantified by dilution of sera.

11.2 Treatment

A two week course of daily procaine penicillin 50,000u/kg or aqueous crystalline penicillin G 50,000u/kg/day in 2 divided doses is recommended, in view of the diagnostic uncertainties of neurosyphilis and poor penicillin penetration into the CSF (McCracken and Kaplan, 1974).

12. Conjunctivitis

Despite its ubiquitous nature and extraordinary prevalence (Elias-Jones et al., 1961; Forfar et al., 1953), neonatal conjunctivitis has attracted little research interest.

12.1 Pathogenic Organisms

The list of accepted pathogens is headed by *Staphylococcus aureus* and Gram-negative enteric bacilli, with the addition of *Neisseria gonorrhoeae* and *Chlamydia trachomatis*. Where practised, Crede's prophylaxis (using 1 % silver nitrate) can be expected to modify the aetiological pattern observed (Armstrong et al., 1976).

Staphylococcus epidermidis is considered normal flora, although the demonstration of toxin producing strains is of interest (Valenton, 1973).

12.2 Diagnosis

Diagnosis is based on cytological and culture examination of the conjunctival exudate. Gram's and Giemsa's stains may permit identification of inflammatory or inclusion-bearing cells (Johnson and Wells, 1971; Goscienski, 1970). The timing of infection and gross nature of the exudate are unreliable guides (Armstrong et al., 1976).

12.3 Treatment

Penicillin is mandatory for proven gonococcal conjunctivitis, and should be given systemically. There are no reports of therapeutic failure, presumably due to high local concentrations. Topical sulphacetamide or tetracycline therapy is effective in inclusion conjunctivitis (Goscienski, 1970); a minimum of two weeks treatment is recommended, with emphasis on careful follow-up examination.

Topical bacitracin is a rational choice for staphylococcal conjunctivitis and neomycin or polymyxin B have proven useful in cases of Gram-negative infection. Locally invasive disease requires systemic therapy. Dacrocystitis responds to massage provided the nasolacrymal duct is patent.

12.4 Prognosis

Prognosis is excellent. Inclusion conjunctivitis can relapse, leading to corneal neovascularisation and scarring. Occlusion of the nasolacrymal duct may be congenital or acquired, and requires surgical probing.

13. Skin Infections

Wound infections, impetigo and Ritter's disease have been discussed in detail in chapter V.

Ritter's form of the 'staphylococcal scalded skin syndrome' may cause diagnostic difficulty unless its toxigenic nature is remembered. Thus Gram stain and culture of the lesions may be negative, as the site of staphylococcal colonisation is often remote (e.g. nares). Fortunately, the differential diagnosis is narrow. Urgent antibiotic therapy is recommended e.g. cloxacillin 200mg/kg/day IV in divided doses 6-hourly.

14. Umbilical Infection

Mild omphalitis continues to be a common problem, but the dreaded complications of fulminant sepsis are now rare. When encountered, purulent umbilical infection is managed by full septic evaluation, debridement and high dose parenteral antibiotic therapy. A Gram smear of the exudate may assist the choice of initial therapy. *Staphylococcus aureus* remains the most common pathogen.

Studies have shown that mixed bacterial colonisation of the umbilicus is universal by the third day (Gunn et al., 1970). Routine skin cleansing with hexachlorophane is no longer recommended; the American Academy of Pediatrics has no alternative suggestion, and is unconvinced of the merits of the procedure (American Academy of Pediatrics, 1972, 1974). Nurseries in Montreal and Toledo have reported reduction in early colonisation with *Staphylococcus aureus* by the use of triple dye applied to the cord stump shortly after birth (Usher, 1975; Katzman, 1975). A group at Stanford have also found topical bacitracin safe and effective (Johnson et al., 1976).

Tetanus neonatorum results from spore contamination of the cord. It persists in under developed countries, where despite aggressive treatment, the disease is fatal in the great majority of cases. Adequate maternal immunisation may provide a measure of transplacental immunity to the newborn.

References

Abbott, G.D.: Transient asymptomatic bacteriuria in infancy. British Medical Journal 1: 207 (1970).

Adler, S.M. and Denton, R.L.: The erythrocyte sedimentation rate in the newborn period. Journal of Pediatrics 86: 942 (1975).

Albers, W.H.; Tyler, C.W. and Boxerman, B.: Asymptomatic bacteremia in the newborn infant. Journal of Pediatrics 69: 193 (1966).

American Academy of Pediatrics (Committee on the Fetus and Newborn): Hexachlorophene. Pediatrics 49: 625 (1972).

American Academy of Pediatrics (Committee on the Fetus and Newborn): Skin care of newborn. Pediatrics 54: 682 (1974).

Armstrong, J.H.; Zacarias, F. and Rein, M.F.: Opthalmia neonatorum: A chart review. Pediatrics 57: 884 (1976).

Baker, C.J.; Barrett, F.F.; Gordon, R.C. and Yow, M.D.: Suppurative meningitis due to streptococci of Lancefield Group B: A study of 33 infants. Journal of Pediatrics 82: 774 (1973).

Barlow, B.; Santulli, T.V.; Heird, W.C.; Pitt, J.; Blanc, W.A. and Schullinger, J.N.: An experimental study of acute neonatal enterocolitis — the importance of breast milk. Journal of Pediatric Surgery 9: 587 (1974).

Barter, R.A. and Hudson, J.A.: Bacteriological findings in perinatal pneumonia. Pathology 6: 223 (1974).

Barton, L.L.; Feigin, R.D. and Lins, R.: Group B beta haemolytic streptococcal meningitis in children. Journal of Pediatrics 82: 719 (1973).

Bell, W.E. and McCormick, W.F.: Neonatal meningitis; in Neurologic Infections in Infants and Children (Saunders, Philadelphia 1975).

Bergstrom, T.; Larson, H.; Lincoln, K. and Winberg, J.: Studies in urinary tract infection in infancy and childhood. 8. Journal of Pediatrics 80: 858 (1972).

Bergstrom, T.; Lincoln, K.; Redin, B. and Winberg, J.: Studies of urinary tract infections in infancy and childhood. 10. Acta Paediatrica Scandinavica 57: 186 (1968).

Bishop, R.F.; Hewstone, A.S.; Davidson, G.P.; Townley, R.R.W.; Holmes, I.H. and Ruck, B.J.: An epidemic of diarrhoea in human neonates involving a reovirus-like agent and 'enteropathogenic' serotypes of Escherichia coli. Journal of Clinical Pathology 29: 46 (1976).

Blanc, W.A.: Pathways of fetal and early neonatal infections. Journal of Pediatrics 59: 473 (1961).

Boyer, K.M.; Peterson, N.J.; Farzaneh, I.; Pattison, C.P.; Hart, M.C. and Maynard, J.E.: An outbreak of gastroenteritis due to E. coli 0142 in a neonatal nursery. Journal of Pediatrics 86: 919 (1975).

Braude, H.; Forfar, J.O.; Gould, J.C. and McLeod, J.W.: Cell and bacterial counts in the urine of normal infants and children. British Medical Journal 4: 697 (1967).

Broughton, D.D.; Mitchell, W.G.; Grossman, M.; Hadley, W.K. and Cohen, M.S.: Recurrence of group B streptococcal infection. Journal of Pediatrics 89: 183 (1976).

Chow, A.; Hecht, R. and Winters, R.: Gentamicin and carbenicillin penetration into the septic joint. New England Journal of Medicine 285: 178 (1971).

De, S.N.; Bhattacharya, K. and Sarkar, J.K.: A study of the pathogenicity of strains of Bacterium coli from acute and chronic enteritis. Journal of Pathology and Bacteriology 71: 201 (1956).

Echeverria, P.; Blocklow, N.R. and Smith, D.H.: Role of heat-labile toxigenic Escherichia coli and reovirus-like agent in diarrhea in Boston children. Lancet 2: 1113 (1975).

Elias-Jones, T.F.; Gordon, I. and Whittaker, L.: Staphylococcal infection of the newborn in hospital and in domicilary practice. British Medical Journal 1: 571 (1961).

Feigin, R.D.: The perinatal group B streptococcal problem: More questions than answers. New England Journal of Medicine 294: 106 (1976).

Forfar, J.O.; Balf, C.L.; Elias-Jones, T.F. and Edmunds, P.N.: Staphylococcal infections of the newborn. British Medical Journal 2: 170 (1953).

Garrod, L.P. and O'Grady, F.: in Antibiotics and Chemotherapy, 3rd Ed. (Churchill Livingstone, London 1972).

Goldman, A.S. and Wayne Smith, C.: Host resistance factors in human milk. Journal of Pediatrics 82: 1082 (1973).

Gorbach, S.L. and Khurana, C.M.: Toxigenic Escherichia coli: A cause of infantile diarrhea in Chicago. New England Journal of Medicine 287: 791 (1972).

Goscienski, P.J.: Inclusion conjunctivitis in the newborn infant. Journal of Pediatrics 77: 19 (1970).

Gotoff, S.P.: Neonatal immunity. Journal of Pediatrics 85: 149 (1974).

Gotoff, S.P. and Behrman, R.E.: Neonatal septicemia. Journal of Pediatrics 76: 142 (1970).

Gunn, G.C.; Mishell, D.R. and Morton, D.G.: Premature rupture of the fetal membranes. American Journal of Obstetrics and Gynecology 106: 469 (1970).

Howard, J.B. and McCracken, G.H.: The spectrum of group B streptococcal infections in infancy. American Journal of Diseases of Children 128: 815 (1974).

Iyengar, L. and Selvaray, R.J.: Intestinal absorption of immunoglobulins by newborn infants. Archives of Diseases in Childhood 47: 411 (1972).

Jawetz, E.: Assay of antibacterial activity in serum. American Journal of Diseases in Children 103: 113 (1962).

Johnson, A.H. and Wells, J.A.: The Gram stain in eye infections. Southern Medical Journal 64: 702 (1971).

Johnson, J.D.; Malachowski, N.C.; Vosti, K.L. and Sunshine, P.: A sequential study of various modes of skin and umbilical care and the incidence of staphylococcal colonization and infection in the neonate. Pediatrics 58: 354 (1976).

Kaiser, A.B. and McGee, Z.A.: Aminoglycoside therapy of Gram-negative bacillary meningitis. New England Journal of Medicine 293: 1215 (1975).

Kapikian, A.Z.; Kim, H.W.; Wyatt, R.G.; Cline, W.L.; Arrobio, J.O; Brandt, C.D.; Rodiguez, W.J.; Sack, D.A.; Chanock, R.M. and Parrott, R.H.: Human reovirus-like agent as the major pathogen associated with winter gastroenteritis in hospitalized infants and young children. New England Journal of Medicine 294: 965 (1976).

Katzman, G.H.: Effects of triple dye in a staphylococcal outbreak. Journal of Pediatrics 86: 313 (1975).

Kincaid-Smith, P. and Fairley, R.F.: Controlled trial comparing effect of two weeks and six weeks treatment in recurrent urinary tract infections. British Medical Journal 2: 145 (1969).

Klastersky, J.; Daneua, D.; Swings, G. and Weerts, D.: Antibacterial activity in serum and urine as a therapeutic guide in bacterial infections. Journal of Infectious Diseases 129: 187-193 (1974).

Kunin, C.M.: Urinary tract infections in infancy. Journal of Pediatrics 86: 483 (1975).

Lincoln, K. and Weinberg, J.: Studies of urinary tract infections in infancy and childhood. 2. Acta Paediatrica Scandinavica 53: 307 (1964).

Littlewood, J.M.: White cells and bacteriuria in voided urine of healthy newborns. Archives of Diseases in Childhood 46: 167 (1971).

Littlewood, J.M.; Kite, P. and Kite, B.A.: Incidence of neonatal urinary tract infection. Archives of Diseases in Childhood 44: 617 (1969).

Lorber, J. and Pickering, D.: Incidence and treatment of post-meningitic hydrocephalus in the newborn. Archives of Diseases in Childhood 41: 44 (1966).

McCracken, G.H.: The rate of bacteriologic response to antimicrobial therapy in neonatal meningitis. American Journal of Diseases in Children 123: 547 (1972).

McCracken, G.H.: Neonatal group B streptococcal infections — editorial comment. Journal of Pediatrics 89: 203 (1976).

McCracken, G.H. and Kaplan, J.M.: Penicillin treatment for congenital syphilis. Journal of the American Medical Association 228: 855 (1974).

McCracken, G.H. and Mize, S.G.: A controlled study of intrathecal antibiotic therapy in Gram-negative enteric meningitis of infancy. Journal of Pediatrics 89: 66 (1976).

Mimica, I.; Donoso, E.; Howard, J.E. and Lederman, G.W.: Lung puncture in the etiological diagnosis of pneumonia; a study of 543 infants and children. American Journal of Diseases in Children 122: 278 (1971).

Moellering, R.C.; Medoff, G.; Leech, I.; Wennersten, C. and Kunz, L.J.: Antibiotic synergism against *Listeria monocytogenes*. Antimicrobial Agents and Chemotherapy 1: 30 (1972).

Murphy, A.M.; Albery, M.B. and Hay, P.J.: Rotavirus infections in neonates. Lancet 2: 452 (1975).

Nelson, J.D.: Duration of neomycin therapy for enteropathogenic *Escherichia coli* diarrheal disease: A comparative study of 113 cases. Pediatrics 48: 248 (1971a).

Nelson, J.D.: Antibiotic concentrations in septic joint effusions. New England Journal of Medicine 284: 349 (1971b).

Nelson, J.D.: The bacterial etiology and antibiotic management of septic arthritis in infants and children. Pediatrics 50: 437 (1972).

Ogden, J.A. and Lister, G.: The pathology of neonatal osteomyelitis. Pediatrics 55: 474 (1975).

Pittard, W.B.; Thullen, J.D. and Fanaroff, A.A.: Neonatal septic arthritis. Journal of Pediatrics 88: 621 (1976).

Pai, C.H.: Personal communication (1976).

Ray, C.G. and Wedgewood, R.J.: Neonatal listerosis. Pediatrics 34: 378 (1964).

Salmon, J.H.: Ventriculitis complicating meningitis. American Journal of Diseases in Children 124: 35 (1972).

Saxena, S.R.; Laurance, B.U. and Shaw, D.G.: The justification for early radiological investigations of urinary tract infection in children. Lancet 2: 403 (1976).

Scanlon, J.: Early recognition of neonatal sepsis. Clinical Pediatrics 11: 258 (1972).

Smith, C.B.; Dans, P.E.; Wilfert, J.N. and Finland, M.: Use of gentamicin in combinations with other antibiotics. Journal of Infectious Diseases 119: 370 (1969).

Stoliar, O.A.; Pelley, R.P.; Kaniecki-Green, E.; Klaus, M.H. and Carpenter, C.C.J.: Secretory IgA against enterotoxins in breast milk. Lancet 1: 1258 (1976).

Usher, R.H.: Personal communications (1975).

Valenton, M.J.: Toxin producing strains of *Staphylococcus epidermidis* isolated from patients with staphylococcal blepharoconjunctivitis. Archives of Ophthalmology 89: 186 (1973).

Vollman, J.H.; Smith, W.L.; Ballard, E.T. and Light, I.J.: Early onset group B streptococcal disease: Clinical roentgenographic, and pathologic features. Journal of Pediatrics 89: 199 (1976).

Weissberg, E.D.; Smith, A.L. and Smith, D.H.: Clinical features of neonatal osteomyelitis. Pediatrics 53: 505 (1974).

Wright, W.C.; Ank, B.J.; Herbert, J. and Stiehm, E.R.: Decreased bactericidal activity of leukocytes of stressed newborn infants. Pediatrics 56: 579 (1975).

Zipursky, A.; Palko, J.; Milner, R. and Akenzua, G.I.: The hematology of bacterial infections in premature infants. Pediatrics 57: 839 (1976).

Subject Index

A